Ethics in Nursing

Ethics in Nursing

Martin Benjamin   Joy Curtis

New York   Oxford
OXFORD UNIVERSITY PRESS
1981

Library of Congress Cataloging in Publication Data
Benjamin, Martin.
  Ethics in nursing.
  Bibliography: p.
  Includes index.
  1. Nursing ethics. I. Curtis, Joy. II. Title.
[DNLM: 1. Ethics, Nursing. WY 85 B468e]
RT85.B39   174'.2   81-511
ISBN 0-19-502836-8   AACR2
ISBN 0-19-502837-6 (pbk.)

Printing (last digit): 987654321
Printed in the United States of America

Preface

The aim of this book is to provide practicing and student nurses with an introduction to the identification and analysis of ethical issues that reflects both the special perspective of nursing and the value of systematic philosophical inquiry. Discussions of general and theoretical points are, wherever possible, grounded in and illustrated by their application to specific nursing situations. The text includes thirty actual cases which are discussed in some detail. In addition, Appendix D contains a set of eleven case studies for further practice in ethical analysis and reasoning.

The book begins with an account of the nature of moral dilemmas and outlines the philosophical skills and understanding necessary for addressing them systematically. Next, Chapter 2 provides an introduction to basic ethical principles and the complex relationships between ethical, legal, and religious considerations in the nursing context. Then, through a series of ten case studies, Chapter 3 focuses upon ethical issues involving nurses and clients. Chapter 4 discusses complications that arise due to the unclear nature of the relationship between nurses and physicians. In Chapter 5 we turn to ethical dilemmas involving relationships among nurses. Finally, Chapter 6 examines the extent to which nurses ought to be concerned with the nature and direction of institutional and public policy.

Throughout the book our emphasis in discussing individual cases is to illustrate the application of ethical analysis and reasoning and the importance of thinking for oneself. Where we come to conclusions on particular points,

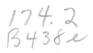

therefore, we do not intend readers to accept them without carefully examining our reasoning. The importance of critically analyzing the reasons given for various positions applies to our arguments no less than to those of others. Readers may or may not agree with our analyses of particular cases, but if they come to their conclusions by applying some of the methods, principles, and distinctions that we have stressed, our purpose will have been fulfilled. As a recent report on *The Teaching of Ethics in Higher Education* put it: "The test of the teaching of ethics is not whether students end by sharing the convictions of their teachers, but whether they have come to those convictions by means of the use of skills that might have led in other directions and may do so in the future" (Hastings-on-Hudson, The Hastings Center, 1980, p. 61).

Unless otherwise noted, all cases presented in the text were obtained from practicing nurses as part of a 1978 research study on nurses' perceptions of ethical dilemmas. The study was based upon one-hour, structured, tape recorded interviews with a sample of forty practicing baccalaureate educated nurses in Michigan's lower peninsula. The distribution of the principal employment settings of the nurses who participated in the study closely approximated the percentage distribution of all active registered nurses in Michigan whose highest degree was in baccalaureate nursing: there were 28 hospital nurses, 5 community health nurses, 3 nursing school faculty, 2 school nurses, 1 nursing home nurse, 1 office nurse, and no private duty, occupational health, or self-employed nurses. While the cases developed from these interviews do not raise all possible ethical issues in nursing, they offer a fair sampling of the ethical dilemmas that frequently recur in nursing practice. Names and places have been changed to insure confidentiality but, wherever possible, the nurses' actual words have been retained.

We want to express our gratitude to the nurses who participated in this study as well as to a number of others who helped us in preparing this book. Isabelle K. Payne, Dean of the College of Nursing at Michigan State University, and Suzanne Brouse, Maureen Chojnacki, Marilyn Rothert, and Linda Beth Tiedje read the manuscript and made suggestions about the nursing aspects. Lewis Zerby and Thomas Tomlinson, of the Department of Philosophy, suggested helpful changes with regard to the philosophical aspects. Linda Henlotter, a graduate assistant in the College of Nursing, helped conduct the interviews of practicing nurses and Stanley Werne, a graduate assistant in the Department of Philosophy, helped compile the list of further readings and made suggestions about the manuscript. Though they are too numerous to mention by name, we also want to express our thanks to students in our team-taught course in Ethics in Nursing who helped us evaluate the clarity and relevance of the manuscript and encouraged us to complete it.

We are grateful, too, to Michigan State University for an M.S.U. Foundation Grant, which supported the survey of nurses, and an All-University Research Grant, which helped in the preparation of the manuscript. Finally, thanks are due to three people who provided special assistance. JoAnn Wittick, of the Medical Humanities Program, cheerfully and skillfully typed the manuscript. Bruce Curtis, of the Department of American Thought and Language, made line by line stylistic improvements. And Jeffrey House, of Oxford University Press, offered detailed criticisms and useful suggestions which helped us strengthen some of our arguments and made certain sections clearer and more concise.

East Lansing, Michigan   M. B.
January, 1981   J.C.

Contents

Cases

Ethics in Nursing

1

Moral Dilemmas and Ethical Inquiry

1. Moral dilemmas in nursing

Advances in medical knowledge and technology, together with social and political changes, have raised a number of well-publicized moral dilemmas for patients and physicians. Less well publicized, but no less important, are the troubling conflicts of value that arise for nurses in these changing circumstances. As an example of the sort of dilemma created by the special role and responsibilities of nursing, consider the following case.

1.1 Truthfulness in terminal illness

Sue Cort, a new staff nurse with over three years of oncological experience in another hospital, was assigned primary responsibility for Ann Haroldson, a recent divorcée in her mid-forties, who had just been diagnosed as having cancer of the colon with metastasis involving lymph nodes. Sue had cared for Mrs. Haroldson for three days preoperatively and had established good rapport with her. Mrs. Haroldson's heavy sedation immediately after surgery plus Sue's being off duty the next day prevented communication between the two until the second postoperative day.

That day it soon became apparent to Sue that Mrs. Haroldson had not been informed about the nature or seriousness of her illness. Thus, her initial response to the patient's inquiries about test results and when she would be able to return to work was judiciously vague. Shortly thereafter, one of Mrs.

3

Haroldson's daughters approached Sue and urged her to assure her mother that there was nothing to be concerned about. Mrs. Haroldson had just gone through a long and unpleasant divorce, she explained, and she and her sister wanted their mother spared the further pain of learning that she had a terminal illness.

Deeply troubled, Sue discussed this situation with her head nurse, who suggested she pursue the matter with Mrs. Haroldson's physician as soon as possible. When she found Dr. Bannister at the nurses' station, Sue indicated that she was caring for Mrs. Haroldson and said that she wanted to know what she had been told about her condition so that she might be more open and supportive with her. She also mentioned the patient's request for information about her condition and intimated that, based on her knowledge of the patient, she thought that Mrs. Haroldson's request was authentic and that she could handle the truth.

In response, Dr. Bannister, who was not Mrs. Haroldson's longstanding physician, said that the patient had not been informed that she had cancer in order to spare her unnecessary anxiety. Moreover, he added, any act of disclosure on the nurse's part would have to be considered inconsistent with the well-being of the patient and inconsistent with her role as a nurse. The general tone of Dr. Bannister's response, though not hostile, was self-assured and disapproving.

Sue then related this to the head nurse and sought her counsel. After acknowledging that Dr. Bannister's position presented Sue with a serious dilemma, she advised her to comply with his directions in order to avoid a messy confrontation. If this sort of thing really bothered her, the head nurse added, she would in the future do what she would to reduce the number of times Sue was assigned to care for one of Dr. Bannister's patients.[1]

In this case the nurse faces a difficult moral dilemma. Strictly speaking, a *dilemma* is a situation requiring a choice between what seem to be two equally desirable or undesirable alternatives. Students sometimes find themselves in a dilemma when they have to choose between two highly rated, interesting courses that are scheduled at the same time. Or one might face a dilemma in deciding whether to go out in the rain to bring in a bicycle or to let it become a bit more rusty: neither alternative, getting wet or the bike's getting rusty, is desirable, but there is no way to avoid both. These, however, are not *moral* dilemmas. In a moral dilemma, *each* alternative course of action can be justified by fundamental moral rules or principles. The nurse who believes that she is duty-bound *both* to preserve life and to reduce suffering may be confronted with a dilemma when preserving life involves prolonging suffering or when suffering cannot be reduced without increasing the likelihood of shortening life. Choosing either seems to violate an ethical principle, yet the choice must be made.

The moral dilemma in "Truthfulness in Terminal Illness" centers on the choice Sue Cort must make between responding in a supportive but nonetheless truthful way to Mrs. Haroldson's questions about her condition or continuing to deflect these questions and assuring her that there is nothing to worry about. On the face of it, each course of action could be grounded on fundamental principles.

A truthful response could be defended by appealing to Mrs. Haroldson's right, as a competent adult, to an honest answer to her questions. This right, it may be argued, is based on the right to self-determination, which is itself based on the respect owed to all persons by virtue of their capacity for choice and reflection. The violation of this right would therefore constitute a significant assault on Mrs. Haroldson's freedom and dignity as a person. Moreover, Sue Cort could also maintain that her participation in the deception seriously compromises the integrity of the relationship between her and the patient, thus diminishing her personhood as well as Mrs. Haroldson's.

On the other hand, acting in accord with the wishes of the family and the physician could also be supported by an appeal to moral principle. Mrs. Haroldson's daughters argue that deception is necessary to spare their mother further pain, and Dr. Bannister says that he wants to spare Mrs. Haroldson unnecessary anxiety. The reduction of pain and suffering is not only a general moral imperative; it has been a cornerstone of both medical and nursing morality. Perhaps this is what Dr. Bannister has in mind when he says that any act of disclosure on Ms. Cort's part would be inconsistent with her role as a nurse. This, too, can be construed as a moral appeal if we assume that Ms. Cort has some sort of moral obligation to the profession and the hospital, as well as to the patient, to act in accord with the special role she has voluntarily assumed.

How, then, should the nurse resolve the dilemma? Perhaps her initial inclination to answer the patient's questions truthfully can no longer be defended. After all, can she disregard the wishes of both the family and the physician? They seem as concerned with the patient's well-being as she is. If she still has some reservations, perhaps the wise thing to do is to take the head nurse's advice and try to avoid such situations in the future, but to go along in this instance. But what if she is right, after all, and they, though well-intentioned, are wrong? If so, wouldn't it be either immoral or cowardly of a nurse not to fulfill her moral obligation to Mrs. Haroldson?

What can Sue Cort appeal to in making her decision? Many people think that codes of medical or nursing ethics should be able to resolve such problems. In the next section we will see to what extent this is so.

2. Ethical codes: uses and limitations

Codes of professional ethics are often a mixture of creeds and commandments. As creeds, they affirm professional regard for high ideals of conduct and personally commit members of the profession to honor them, thus constituting a sort of oath of professional office. The opening sentence of the 1973 Code for Nurses of the International Council of Nurses (Appendix A) states that "The fundamental responsibility of the nurse is fourfold: to promote health, to prevent illness, to restore health and to alleviate suffering." This is a statement of creed. As commandments, codes of professional ethics provide a set of prescriptions designed to regulate conduct in more specific situations. For example, the same International Council of Nurses' Code states that "The Nurse holds in confidence personal information and uses judgement in sharing this information."

As creeds, codes of nursing ethics provide a valuable reminder of the special responsibilities incumbent upon those who tend the sick. Nurses often deal with people who, because of their illness or injury, are especially vulnerable and must depend upon the professional's special knowledge and skills. Hence, it is important that the nursing profession formulate and adhere to high ideals of conduct in order to assure the public that individual nurses will not exploit their advantaged positions.

As sets of commandments, codes of professional ethics have two principal functions. First, they provide an enforceable standard of minimally decent conduct that allows the profession to discipline those who clearly fall below the minimal standard. For example, in 1978 the *New Yorker* reported that some nurses were being paid by antiabortion groups for the names of women who had had abortions. Members of these groups then proceeded to harass the women with abusive phone calls when they returned from the hospital.[2] Such conduct on the part of the nurses in question, regardless of the strength or correctness of their views on abortion, clearly violates both the provision of the International Council's Code stating that "The Nurse holds in confidence personal information and uses judgement in sharing this information" and Point 2 of the 1976 American Nurses' Association Code for Nurses (Appendix B) which holds that "The nurse safeguards the client's right to privacy by judiciously protecting information of a confidential nature."

A second function of the commandments in codes of professional ethics is to indicate in general terms some of the ethical considerations professionals must take into account in deciding on conduct. Thus, as indicated above, privacy and confidentiality are important considerations. So too are maintaining one's own professional competence and safeguarding patients from the incompetent, unethical, or illegal practice of others.

It is a mistake to think that all a conscientious nurse needs in order to deal with the moral dilemmas that arise in nursing is an adequate code of ethics coupled with a healthy measure of common sense. To demonstrate the limitations of ethical codes we need only try to resolve Sue Cort's moral dilemma in "Truthfulness in Terminal Illness" by appealing to the International Council's Code and the American Nurses' Association (ANA) Code.

Parts of the Code for Nurses of the International Council of Nurses can be cited to support each alternative in Sue Cort's dilemma. For example, a decision to respond honestly to Mrs. Haroldson's questions can be based on the provisions of the Code which hold that: "Inherent in nursing is respect for . . . dignity"; "The nurse's primary responsibility is to those people who require nursing care"; "The nurse, in providing care, promotes an environment in which the values, customs and spiritual beliefs of the individual are respected"; and "The nurse carries personal responsibility for nursing practice. . . ." Thus, it could be argued that the Code requires Sue Cort to be truthful with Mrs. Haroldson in order to respect her dignity, beliefs, and values, and because her primary responsibility is to the patient and not to her daughters or to the physician. Moreover, because Sue carries personal responsibility for what she does, she, and not the head nurse or the doctor, must make the final decision.

On the other hand, one can also cite provisions of this Code to support the opposing position. For example, the Code also states that one of the "fundamental responsibilities" of the nurse is "to alleviate suffering"; "The nurse holds in confidence personal information and uses judgement in sharing this information"; and "The nurse sustains a cooperative relationship with co-workers in nursing and other fields." It could, therefore, be argued that the Code requires that Sue Cort not inform Mrs. Haroldson of the nature and seriousness of her condition, since this would create needless suffering, exhibit poor judgment in sharing confidential information, and seriously strain the cooperative relationship she is supposed to sustain with the physician.

To interpret this Code in a way that supports one or the other of Sue Cort's choices would be controversial and would require a considerable amount of supporting argument. Moreover, the usefulness of the Code as a straightforward guide to the resolution of moral dilemmas would be significantly diminished by such interpretations.

The source of the difficulty is not so much this particular code but with the very idea of attempting to codify, in a simple yet consistent and comprehensive way, all of the precepts one needs to resolve dilemmas in a field as morally complex as nursing. Any such attempt will be caught on one of the horns of a difficult dilemma. If the code is to be simple, comprehensive, and acceptable to all nurses, it will be so abstract and general that it cannot, without significant interpretation, be applied to many specific problems. Such codes may gain widespread acceptance before their use in actual situations, but only because their vagueness allows people holding opposing views to mask their differences by interpreting the code in accord with their favored position on various issues. When the code is then appealed to in dilemmas like that facing Sue Cort, the hitherto submerged differences in interpretation rise to the surface and those who are engaged in the dispute must go beyond the code itself in order to resolve them. If, on the other hand, one tries to draft a very specific code aimed at anticipating all of the moral problems that can arise, one encounters three significant problems. First, the code will not be able to avoid controversial precepts and hence will be unlikely to win widespread acceptance. Second, it will probably fill many thick volumes, and thus lose the advantages of brevity and simplicity. And third, no matter how detailed it is, such a code will always be incomplete if its aim is to give unambiguous guidance in all possible situations. Therefore, neither a brief, simple code nor a long, detailed one will both offer clear guidance and attain widespread acceptance.

Before accepting this argument about the limitations of codes of professional ethics, let us briefly examine the 1976 ANA Code for Nurses. As the editors of the *Encyclopedia of Bioethics* have pointed out, this eleven-point Code, together with the interspersed Interpretive Statements that go with it, is distinctive among codes of ethics because:

(1) It identifies the values and beliefs which undergird the ethical standards; (2) it shows a remarkable breadth of social and professional concerns; (3) it manifests an awareness of the ethical implications of shifting professional roles and of the complexity of modern health care; and (4) it goes beyond prescriptive statements regarding personal and professional conduct by advocating a sense of accountability to the client.[3]

One might think, therefore, that if this code cannot unambiguously resolve Sue Cort's dilemma, then it is unlikely that any reasonably simple code *accepted by the nursing profession* will be able to do so—at least in the foreseeable future.

Admirable as the 1976 ANA Code is, when applied to Sue Cort's dilemma, it seems to neutralize at one point what it has affirmed at another. For example, *1.1 Self-Determination of Clients* first states that "Each client has the moral right to determine what will be done with his/her person; to be given the information necessary for making informed judgments; to be told the possible effects of care; and to accept, refuse or terminate treatment." The next paragraph, however, adds that, "The nurse must also recognize those situations in which individual rights to self-determination in health care may temporarily be altered for the common good." Thus, we wonder whether the case of Mrs. Haroldson is one of "those situations" or not. Whatever the answer, it is not to be found in the code itself.

Section *1.6 The Dying Person* is equally ambiguous. The sentence which states that "The nurse seeks ways to protect these [basic human] values while working with the client and others to arrive at the best decisions dictated by the circumstances, the *client's rights and wishes*, and the highest standards of care" (our emphasis) seems to support a decision to tell Mrs. Haroldson about her illness. But the very next sentence, "The measures used to provide assistance should enable the client to live with as much comfort, dignity, and *freedom from anxiety* and pain as possible" (our emphasis) might be used by Mrs. Haroldson's daughters and physician to justify withholding the truth. Again, the code reminds us of relevant values but gives little indication of how to resolve conflicts of values, which are the very stuff of moral dilemmas.

Our aim has not been to belittle the ANA Code—indeed, as codes of professional ethics go, it is among the best—but rather to demonstrate the limitations of any code of professional ethics as a resource for resolving difficult moral dilemmas. That any code will be limited in this way can be explained in part by an examination of the most basic question of philosophical ethics.

3. The fundamental question of morality

Ethics, understood here as a discipline whose roots go back to Socrates, is an attempt to formulate and justify systematic responses to the following question: "What, *all things considered*, ought to be done in a given situation?" It is the unrestricted frame of reference indicated by the phrase "all things considered" that limits the usefulness of ethical codes and makes ethics such a difficult subject.

Many questions about what a person ought to do raise no ethical questions because they are limited to a certain context where a definite framework establishes various rules and roles that provide unambiguous direction. Thus, suppose that a person is playing checkers. At various points in the game she may ask herself, "What should I do?" Assuming that the question is bounded by the rules of the game and motivated by a desire to win, it is not an ethical one. The answer will be determined solely by appeal to the rules and strategies of checkers. Similar questions that arise *within* various clearly defined occupational or familial roles may be answered in the same way. But now suppose that we expand the account of the circumstances of our checker-player to include that her opponent is her five-year-old son, who is just learning the game. Here the question of what move she ought to make in a given situation is more complex. Of course, if she wants to disregard the fact that her opponent is a beginner and her child, she may proceed as before. But if she considers that her opponent is her son and that he is just learning the game, she will want to play with much less competitive vigor than if he were someone like herself. Her task here is a ticklish one. Because she presumably wants to help develop her son's skills and knowledge without crushing his spirit, she must play reasonably well (otherwise he would never learn to play well himself) but not too well (otherwise his confidence would be dealt a severe blow). So, as this simple example shows, determining what one ought to do, *all things considered*, is more complex than determining what one ought to do within a more narrowly circumscribed frame of reference. And as with the combined roles of checker-player and parent, so too there can be tension between what one ought to do as employee, citizen, parent, spouse, etc., where these roles overlap.

Consider, for example, a driver who approaches an intersection at 3:00 A.M. as he is taking his pregnant wife, whose labor has begun, to the hospital. The light is red and there are no other cars in sight. Should he wait until the light turns green or proceed through the intersection? As a law-abiding citizen he has a duty to wait; but as a husband taking his wife to the hospital, it could be argued that he has a duty, after checking for traffic, to continue. Thus, the question arises as to what, all things considered, he ought to do. And this *moral* question requires that the framework of inquiry go beyond a simple appeal to the ordinary requirements of drivers and husbands, respectively.

Ethical issues about whether one ought or ought not to do something arise, then, when a question cannot be answered by appeal to the special or restricted considerations governing clearly defined and justifiable roles or practices. Here one must enlarge the frame of reference and identify and critically examine all the relevant considerations. It is this matter of a completely unrestricted frame of reference that makes ethical inquiry so difficult. The range and complexity of relevant factual and value-laden considerations often outstrip our initial capacity to comprehend and evaluate them. This is especially true of problems that arise within the medical and nursing context. The problems are more difficult now than ever before partly because the complexities of modern medicine have required the development of health care "teams," made up of different sorts of professionals, whose respective roles cannot always be precisely defined. Given the complexity of the clinical encounter and the nature of ethics (with its completely unrestricted frame of reference), no simple code—together with common sense—can relieve the thoughtful health professional of the difficult and demanding task of ethical inquiry. The reflective nurse cannot put her moral course on "automatic pilot."

4. Ethical inquiry

Even if a widely accepted code of ethics could provide unambiguous solutions to moral dilemmas in nursing, we would want to know whether these were the best or most nearly correct solutions and if this were the best code. To answer these questions, we would have to rely on conventional ethical analysis. This same sort of analysis must be applied directly to the dilemmas that resist a codified solution. The first step in this analysis is to identify ethical or other value-laden issues in nursing in this case, and to distinguish them from purely technical or empirical concerns. Next, we use various skills of ethical analysis and reasoning in an attempt to reach a well-grounded solution. At various points in this process, we may also have to consider the nature and limits of ethical knowledge as well as the nature and justification of basic ethical principles.

A. Identification of ethical issues

Health care professionals who are unaware of the value-laden elements of their practice may, in the name of technical expertise, impose their (often unexamined) personal values on others without adequate justification. Once it is recognized, however, that a particular question is not solely—or even mainly—a function of medical or nursing expertise, the health care professional can then try to determine who can best answer it and what, all things considered, seems to be the best grounded solution or range of solutions.

Thus, a decision to withhold the truth cannot, like a decision to intubate, be justified by a physician's appeal to *medical* expertise. If a nurse and a physician disagree over whether a patient should be intubated, surely the presumption must be that the physician, in virtue of his or her more extensive training and knowledge, is correct. But, as Roland R. Yarling has argued:

> Because the question is non-medical in nature, if there is a disagreement between a nurse and a physician about whether a terminal patient who requests the information should be told of his diagnosis and prognosis, the matter of whose opinion should prevail is not clear as it is in the situation where intubation is the question. There, because judgment is nonmedical, the medical expertise of the physician does not give his opinion an extraordinary value. The question whether to inform the terminal patient of his condition is essentially a moral one, and decision on that question is a moral, rather than a medical, decision. This being so, neither the physician, as a physician, nor the nurse, as nurse, may claim a privileged position with respect to making that judgment.[4]

Once an issue is identified as basically a moral or value-laden one, it is appropriate to use the various skills that characterize ethical inquiry to try to reach a well-grounded solution.

B. Ethical analysis and reasoning

Critical reflection and inquiry in ethics involve the complex interplay of a variety of human faculties, ranging from empathy and moral imagination on the one hand to analytic precision and careful reasoning on the other. Among the more cognitive skills one employs in thinking an ethical issue through are the following:

1. Determining and obtaining relevant factual information. Although genuine moral dilemmas cannot be resolved simply by an appeal to or understanding of "the facts," certain factual matters will always be relevant to ethical inquiry. If we must reach beyond the facts in attempting to resolve a moral dilemma, we must also guard against reaching without them. Thus, for example, in "Truthfulness in Terminal Illness," it is important that Sue Cort be very clear about such things as Mrs. Haroldson's prognosis, the authenticity of her request for information, and various other psychosocial and biomedical data.

2. Aiming at conceptual clarity and drawing relevant distinctions. The complexity of ethical inquiry often requires careful conceptual analysis and the recognition of important distinctions. For example, many controversies in health care involve conflicting claims of rights. These include the "right to life," the "right to die," "patient's rights," "society's rights," and "right to one's own body," the "right to health care," and numerous other "rights," all of which are often invoked to support one or another resolution of a moral dilemma. But what, exactly, is a "right"? What, we may ask, does it *mean* to say that people have a "right to life?" Does it mean that it is wrong, under any circumstances (e.g., capital punishment, war, or in self-defense) to kill people? Or that killing is wrong only when it is "unjust" (and how, exactly, do we determine whether a particular killing is "unjust")? In addition, does the "right to life" require that people also be given whatever is necessary to sustain their lives (even if doing so requires enormous expenditures and forces significant reductions in other areas such as education, housing, and treatment for illness and injuries which are not life-threatening)? A satisfactory analysis of the concept of a "right" and of the various "rights" *in* and *to* health care (including the "right to life") is necessary if appeals to "rights" are to play any but a rhetorical role in the resolution of moral dilemmas in medicine and nursing. The same is true of such concepts as "health," "disease," "advocate," "death with dignity," "sanctity of life," "euthanasia," "benefit" and "mental illness." One of the reasons ethical debates often become fruitless and frustrating is that the participants fail to clarify adequately what they are talking about.

The result of a careful conceptual analysis is often the recognition of one or more distinctions that had not previously been explicitly recognized. Drawing an important distinction in ethical inquiry can be likened to using fine instruments in surgery. The surgeon needs very fine instruments to cut or suture one particular part of the body while leaving others untouched. Neither a woodsman's axe nor a kitchen knife is suited for surgical incisions because they are too crude or blunt and will cut far more than should be cut. So too, in ethical inquiry, one needs fine tools to outline a defensible position on one particular issue without thereby being committed, less defensibly, to the same position on a different kind of issue. It is one thing, for example, to argue for allowing conscious, competent, adult Jehovah's Witnesses to refuse lifesaving blood transfusions for themselves and quite another to allow them to do so for their minor children. Our tools here are words; fine linguistic distinctions, like fine surgical instruments, make possible more precise analysis of complex questions.

As an example of conceptual analysis and drawing relevant distinctions, let us briefly examine the notion of a "medical decision." Patients and physicians often invoke the notion of a "medical decision" to justify the physician's authority to make one or another decision in the course of treatment. Many people, for example, might be inclined to support Dr. Bannister's decision to withhold Mrs. Haroldson's diagnosis from her because it is a "medical decision" and he, after all, *is* the doctor. On these grounds, Sue Cort would be overstepping the bounds of her authority by even suggesting a truthful response to Mrs. Haroldson's request for information. But this line of argument reveals some confusion about the concept of "medical decision."

There are two critically different senses in which something may be a "medical decision." In the first, a medical decision is one that is based directly on medical knowledge or expertise. Such decisions are a function of a physician's special training. Let us call such decisions "medical decisions in the technical sense" and identify this use of the term "medical decision" with the subscript "t." Examples of medical decisions$_t$ are decisions about the medical diagnosis and prognosis of a particular illness, the correct dosage of various medications, and how best to perform a certain surgical procedure in a given case.

The term "medical decision" can also be used to refer to any decision made in the medical context. Such decisions, however, are not always a function of medical knowledge or expertise, though they may be informed by them. They will often turn on questions of value, and as we noted above, the physician's technical expertise does not make him or her an expert on conflicts of value. Let us call such decisions "medical decisions in the contextual sense" and identify this use of the term "medical decisions" with the subscript "c." Decisions in health care that are largely a matter of resolving a conflict of values or of other factors that are not exclusively medical will thus be called medical decisions$_c$. These include decisions about whether a patient should be informed of the diagnosis and prognosis of a certain illness; whether the costs, inconvenience, or risks of a certain medication are outweighed by the benefits; and whether, all things considered, a patient should undergo a certain surgical procedure. Having made this distinction, we can say that "Not all medical decisions$_c$ are medical decisions$_t$."

The decision about disclosing Mrs. Haroldson's diagnosis is a medical decision in the contextual sense. The controversy turns largely on a conflict of values and not on matters of medical expertise. To attempt to cut off ethical inquiry by an appeal to the decision's medical nature is to fail to appreciate the distinction between medical decisions$_t$ and medical decisions$_c$. Although this does not show that Sue Cort's inclination to disclose the prognosis to Mrs. Haroldson is correct, it does show that she is not, in pursuing the question, mounting any sort of challenge to Dr. Bannister's expertise *as a physician*. She might be on considerably weaker ground, however, had Dr. Bannister been Mrs. Haroldson's longstanding physician.

3. Constructing and evaluating arguments. We use the word "argument" in the logician's sense, in which an argument is a set of reasons, or premises, together with a claim, or conclusion, which they are intended to support. Having identified an ethical issue, we must not only conduct factual and conceptual investigations; we must also construct and evaluate arguments for and against various positions.

In so doing, we search out reasons for or against a certain position and critically determine the extent to which these reasons, as premises, constitute good grounds for accepting the conclusion. In the case of "Truthfulness in Terminal Illness," for example, Dr. Bannister suggests an argument for his decision to withhold the diagnosis and prognosis from Mrs. Haroldson. The argument, when spelled out, might have two premises, one of which is assumed to be true, although it is not explicitly stated:

1. Telling Mrs. Haroldson the truth will cause her unnecessary anxiety. (This is the stated premise.)
2. One ought to spare patients unnecessary anxiety. (This premise seems to be assumed, but is not stated.)

If Sue Cort is still inclined to question Dr. Bannister's conclusions, she will have to show exactly where and why these reasons fail to support the conclusion that Mrs. Haroldson shouldn't be told the truth.

An argument must meet two principal conditions if its premises are to be regarded as good grounds for accepting the truth of the conclusion. The first has to do with the argument's *validity*. "Validity," as used in logic, is a technical term referring to the logical connection between an argument's premises and conclusion. An argument is valid if the assumption that its premises are true gives us very good grounds for supposing that its conclusion is true. Validity, then, has to do not with the *actual* truth or falsity of the premises, but rather with the logical connection between the premises and the conclusion *if* we suppose that the premises are true. Thus, for example, both of the following arguments are valid, even though the second premise of B is false:

A. 1. All people are mortal
   2. Socrates is a person
   3. Therefore, Socrates is mortal

B. 1. All horses are mortal
   2. Socrates is a horse
   3. Therefore, Socrates is a mortal

Although both A and B are, strictly speaking, valid arguments, B shows that there is more to an argument's providing good grounds for accepting its conclusion than its being valid. The premises of a good argument would not only provide support for the conclusion *if they were true*, but they must also in fact *be true*. A valid argument whose premises are true is called a *sound* argument. Both arguments A and B are valid, but only A is sound. An argument whose premises provide good grounds for accepting its conclusion will be sound as well as valid.

Let us now examine the argument we have attributed to Dr. Bannister for its validity and soundness. First, the argument seems valid. If the premises are true, then the conclusion will be true. But are the premises true? Is the argument sound? It seems to us that the argument we have attributed to Dr. Bannister, though valid, is of questionable soundness.

One can initially challenge both premises of Dr. Bannister's argument. The first premise, at the very least, needs further support. Factual support is needed to show that telling the truth would cause Mrs. Haroldson *more* anxiety than the anxiety she now appears to be experiencing because of her uncertainty and, perhaps, her perception that her physician, family, and nurse are being less than forthright in responding to her queries. Here, of course, questions also arise as to which of the parties, Dr. Bannister, Mrs. Haroldson's daughters, or Sue Cort is most qualified and in the best position to make this judgment. Furthermore, even if she were to experience more anxiety by being told of her condition, it still has to be shown that this is *unnecessary* anxiety. Perhaps, when looking at the larger scheme of things, it could be argued that this anxiety, though regrettable, is, all things considered, unavoidable if certain other important values are to be acknowledged (such as her freedom to make certain plans or decisions about how she wants to spend the remainder of her life). Thus, we need an analysis of the concept of "unnecessary anxiety" and an indication of the criteria to be used in determining whether a certain amount of anxiety is "unnecessary."

The same applies to the second (implied) premise, that "one ought to spare patients unnecessary anxiety." Like premise (1), this rule requires a careful analysis of what can be considered *unnecessary* anxiety. Given the rule's scope, any such analysis will be deeply immersed in value-laden considerations and may, if pursued thoroughly enough, involve an appeal to one's most basic beliefs about the nature and meaning of human existence. And since people's views of the nature and meaning of human existence are not uniform, it is presumptuous to think that the second premise is both clear enough to guide conduct *and* so well accepted that it needs no supporting argument itself. Insofar as it is clear enough to guide conduct in all relevant cases, it will lack widespread acceptance; insofar as it is widely accepted, it will probably be only vaguely understood and will need to be tempered by successive applications to a variety of complex cases.

Our reconstruction and evaluation of Dr. Bannister's argument has shown that it cannot, at this point, be accepted as sound. We have not, however, shown that his conclusion is false—only that the argument he appears to have in mind does not, in its present form, support his conclusion. It is still open to him to reformulate the argument so that the premises do, in fact, provide good grounds for accepting the conclusion. On the other hand, those who want to show not only that his argument is weak but also that his conclusion is false must now attempt to construct a sound argument whose conclusion is something like: "One ought to tell Mrs. Haroldson the truth." A more thorough examination of the sorts of arguments that might be given in this case will be found in the section entitled "Deception" in Chapter 3.

4. Developing a systematic framework.   Efforts to construct and evaluate particular arguments should draw upon and be incorporated into a developing, systematic, ethical framework. The development of such a framework is important for two reasons. First, it provides a common ground for resolving moral disagreements among people. Insofar as we share a systematic framework, made up of principles, rules, distinctions, standards of justification, etc., we will then be able to use it to settle certain disputes. And even in those cases—so frequent in modern health care—in which such a framework gives no direct guidance, it can at least provide a common background and starting point for the development of satisfactory resolutions.

Second, the development of a systematic ethical framework is of personal as well as interpersonal value. One of the qualities most of us admire in others and try to cultivate in ourselves is personal integrity. A person of integrity, in this sense, is one whose responses to various matters are not capricious or arbitrary, but principled. Such a person attempts to respond to new situations, as far as possible, in ways that are consistent with justifiable responses to past situations. This principled continuity of conduct is part of his or her identity as a person, and the degree to which he or she is able to *integrate* responses to various situations determines the extent of his or her integrity and identity as a particular person. Thus, so far as a person wants to maintain a unitary sense of identity and an accompanying sense of personal integrity and reliability, he or she will want to adopt a systematic framework for analyzing and responding to ethical issues.

Given the open-ended nature of the fundamental question of morality ("What, all things considered, ought to be done?") and the complexity of our rapidly changing world (with the special difficulties created by the high stakes, personal intimacy, and enlarged range of possibilities that characterize moral dilemmas in the medical context), the development and maintenance of a personal and interpersonal ethical framework requires continual attention. As an ethical framework is repeatedly applied, tested, refined, and revised, its adequacy is gauged by the extent to which it is consistent, coherent, and comprehensive.

An ethical framework is *consistent* to the extent that its particular judgments, rules, and principles are logically compatible and do not contradict one another. A particularly bald example of inconsistency in an ethical framework appears in a widely reprinted article on "Moral and Ethical Dilemmas in the Special-Care Nursery."[5] In discussing the reluctance of specialists in newborn intensive care to deal with issues having to do with conflict between parents and physicians over discontinuing treatment, the authors write: "Some physicians recognize that the wishes of the families went against their own, but they were resolute [about continuing treatment]. They commonly agreed that if they were the parents of very defective children, withholding treatment would be most desirable for them. However, they argued aggressive management was indicated for others" (p. 892). Unless these physicians can justifiably demonstrate a morally relevant difference between themselves *as parents* and the parents of their patients, their ethical frameworks are inconsistent. Other things being equal, if aggressive management is indicated for others, it is indicated for oneself; and if withholding treatment is desirable for oneself as a parent, why is it not desirable for other parents?

An ethical system is *coherent* insofar as its individual judgments, rules, and principles are mutually supportive. The elements of a coherent framework "hang together" so that it provides a systematic basis for addressing unprecedented dilemmas. Controversy over the use of life-prolonging medical technology, for example, might be more readily resolved by appeal to a set of rules and principles that are themselves related to widely accepted judgments about prolonging life in less controversial contexts.

It is often tempting to obtain both consistency and coherence for an ethical framework by restricting its domain or *comprehensiveness*. If consistency has to do with logical compatibility and coherence with mutual support, both will be easier to achieve and maintain within a restricted frame of reference. But to do so would be to retreat from one of the aims of systematic ethical inquiry: the development of a comprehensive framework that will provide guidance in all contexts of moral choice. Other things being equal, then, the wider the range of situations in which a framework is able to provide systematic (i.e., consistent and coherent) guidance, the better it is.

Although consistency, coherence, and comprehensiveness are all important criteria for the adequacy of an ethical framework, people sometimes over-emphasize one at the expense of the others. A restricted definition of "medical ethics," for instance, encompassing only the decisions of doctors, might make it easier to construct a consistent framework. To the extent that many of the most important ethical questions arising in health care require decisions by patients, health planners, citizens, and other health professionals, however, the framework would lack both coherence and comprehensiveness.

5. Anticipating and Responding to Objections. No matter how careful our ethical analysis has been, it is always possible that our reasoning was defective, that we overlooked some important factor, or that new social or biomedical developments have undermined some of our basic assumptions. We must therefore be concerned not only with critically evaluating the positions of others, but also with anticipating and responding to possible objections to our own position and arguments. As John Stuart Mill argues in his celebrated essay *On Liberty*:

> He who knows only his own side of the case knows little of that. His reasons may be good, and no one may have been able to refute them. But if he is equally unable to refute the reasons on the opposite side, if he does not so much as know what they are, he has no ground for preferring either opinion. . . . Ninety-nine in a hundred of what are called educated men are in this condition, even of those who can argue fluently for their opinions. Their conclusion may be true, but it might be false for anything they know; they have never thrown themselves into a mental position of those who think differently from them, and considered what such persons may have to say; and, consequently, they do not, in any proper sense of the word, know the doctrine which they themselves profess. . . . So essential is this discipline to a real understanding of moral and human subjects that, if opponents of all-important truths do not exist, it is indispensable to imagine them and supply them with the strongest arguments which the most skillful devil's advocate can conjure up.[6]

C. Ethical principles and knowledge

In addition to skills in ethical analysis and reasoning, ethical inquiry often requires an understanding of the nature and justification of basic ethical principles, the status of knowledge in ethics, and the relationships among ethics, law, and religion. These very complex topics will be examined in the next chapter. What follows is simply a brief introduction to each area in order to complete our overview of ethical inquiry.

1. Basic ethical principles. Suppose Sue Cort and Dr. Bannister agree, after some discussion, that the question of whether to tell Mrs. Haroldson the truth is a moral and not a purely medical matter. Suppose, too, that they agree on the facts (including the prediction that the longer Mrs. Haroldson remains ignorant of the true state of affairs, the happier she will be—in the ordinary sense of "happy"), and that they are using words in the same way. In these circumstances it is still possible for Ms. Cort and Dr. Bannister to disagree, if, for example, the principle of utility is the foundation of his ethical framework while she espouses some version of the Kantian notion of respect for personal autonomy and dignity as the basic principle of ethics.

Appealing to the utilitarian imperative to maximize the general happiness, Dr. Bannister may reason that not informing Mrs. Haroldson will, on balance, bring about more happiness than unhappiness and that therefore she should not be informed about her condition. Ms. Cort, on the other hand, may argue that preserving a person's autonomy and dignity is more important from a moral point of view than maximizing his or her happiness. Since withholding the truth both restricts Mrs. Haroldson's autonomy and violates her dignity as a self-determining person, Ms. Cort would argue that the patient ought to be told the truth even if this limits her happiness. If the disagreement between Ms. Cort and Dr. Bannister takes this form, there is no way to resolve it apart from examining the nature and justification of the principle of utility and the principle of respect for persons and attempting to determine which principle is most basic in cases in which they give conflicting direction.

2. *Knowledge in ethics.* How do we determine whether one or another proposal for a basic ethical principle is better grounded than the others? This requires some understanding of ethical principles and the way they are organized into ethical frameworks, which equips us to identify and defend our criteria for determining that one of these theories or frameworks is more adequate than the others. To do this we must know, in turn, something about the extent to which ethics is a cognitive discipline. Many people believe it is impossible to show that one framework is more adequate than another because there is no such thing as knowledge in ethics. Moral judgments, they maintain, are neither true nor false, but rather "subjective," nothing more than expressions of personal preference or taste. If this were correct, our efforts to resolve moral dilemmas and disagreements rooted in differences of basic principles would be pointless. So it is vital to refute this popular, skeptical challenge to the possibility of knowledge in ethics (see Chapter 2).

3. *Ethics, law, and religion.* Legal and religious considerations may be relevant in various ways to the resolution of moral dilemmas. But how are they relevant and how much weight are they to be given in various contexts?

To what extent, for example, can Sue Cort, Mrs. Haroldson's daughters, or Dr. Bannister appeal to the law to support their respective positions? If something is illegal, is it also necessarily unethical? And if something is not illegal, does it follow that it is morally permissible? Some understanding of the relationships between legal and ethical considerations is necessary for ethical inquiry.

So too is an understanding of the relationships between religious and ethical considerations. For we may ask to what extent, if any, are ethical claims grounded upon, and inseparable from, religious ones? And to what extent must an acceptable ethical framework allow for decisions based on appeals to religious conviction?

5. Ethical autonomy and institutional-hierarchical constraints

Generally speaking, individuals are autonomous to the extent that they are self-determining or able to act in accord with a plan they had either freely chosen or at least independently endorsed. In everyday life, personal autonomy is a function of the degree to which one can be regarded as *one's own person*, capable of independent action and judgment. By regarding autonomy as a matter of degree, we suggest that people can be *more* or *less* autonomous than others as well as more autonomous in one area of their lives and less in another. Thus, for example, Ann can be regarded as more autonomous than Bea, but less than Celia; and she can be more autonomous as a teacher than she is as a wife or mother.

Ethical autonomy has a central place in the network of moral concepts and is closely related to the notions of personhood, self-respect, and moral responsibility. In fact it is unlikely that a satisfactory analysis of any of these concepts can avoid referring to the others. Ethical autonomy involves being one's own person when one decides upon or judges conduct. To the extent that someone is not her own person, her will becomes the instrument of another or she may be a "cog in a machine." To be seen in this way is to fail to be respected as a person. Respect for persons, Kant pointed out, involves their being regarded as *ends-in-themselves*, not as mere means to someone else's ends. To be an end-in-oneself is to be capable of independent thought and action. Thus, the choices, commitments, and projects of an end-in-herself are worthy of respect not because they produce good results but because they *are* the choices, commitments, and projects of a person. To have self-respect in this context is simply to respect oneself *as a person*, as a being capable of deliberation on ethical questions and one whose choices and decisions, when effected, will result in certain changes in the world. In the ethical sphere, then, self-respect includes holding oneself morally responsible for the results of one's choices and decisions. We may summarize this extremely brief account by stating that to respect oneself (and be respected) as a person it is necessary to cultivate one's ethical autonomy and thus increase the range of things for which one is morally responsible.

A special problem, however, arises for nurses. Put bluntly it is this: To what extent can a nurse be ethically autonomous? Consider, for example, this view of the primary role of a nurse:

> In my estimation obedience is the first law and the very cornerstone of good nursing. And here is the first stumbling block for the beginner. No matter how gifted she may be, she will never become a reliable nurse until she can obey without question. The first and most helpful criticism I ever received from a doctor was when he told me that I was supposed to be simply an intelligent machine for the purpose of carrying out his orders.[7]

Good nursing and ethical autonomy are, according to this writer, incompatible.

Although the author of this passage is reported to have been "a considerable influence on nursing in her time,"[8] that time was over 70 years ago, and her position would probably be met with disbelief or scorn if propounded to contemporary nurses. Yet the behavior it urges nurses to adopt may to a large extent remain even when exhortations to practice it have become embarassing. In 1966, for example, a study of nurse-physician relationships revealed that nurses often complied with medical directives that they knew fell short of minimally decent standards of practice.[9] The researchers structured a situation in which a doctor directed a nurse to administer a particular dose of medication. The directive was unusual because the dosage of medication was obviously excessive; the directive was transmitted by telephone, which violated hospital policy, and the voice was one with which the nurse would not be familiar; and the medication was unauthorized inasmuch as it had not been placed on the ward stock list. Nonetheless, the study showed that twenty one out of a sample of twenty two nurses placed in this situation prepared the medication and were set to give it to the patient when the researchers finally intervened.

This study bears on our present concerns in two ways. First, it shows that some degree of ethical autonomy is a desirable characteristic in a nurse *as a nurse*. As the authors of the study state:

> In a real-life situation corresponding to the experimental one, there would in theory be two professional intelligences, the doctor's and the nurse's, working to ensure that a given procedure be undertaken in a manner beneficial to the patient or, at the very

least, not detrimental to him. The experiment strongly suggests, however, that in the real-life situation one of these intelligences is, for all practical purposes, non-functioning.[10]

Secondly, the study obviously indicates that there may be a discrepancy between a nurse's professed ethical autonomy and the actual nature of her behavior in situations where its exercise involves possible conflicts with physicians, hospitals, or others presumed to have some authority. The researchers observe that

In nonstressful moments, when thinking about her performance, the average nurse tends to believe that considerations of her patient's welfare and of her own professional honor will outweigh considerations leading to automatic obedience to the doctor's orders at times when these two sets of factors come into conflict.[11]

The nursing context is characterized by a number of constraints that frequently make the exercise of autonomy problematic. Over 75 percent of nurses must contend not only with the conventional hierarchical structure of medical decision-making but also with restrictions on behavior imposed by the bureaucratic system of the hospital. Thus, the hospital nurse finds herself constrained in various and occasionally conflicting ways by the hospital (which employs her), the physician (with whom she works), the client (for whom she provides care), and the nursing profession (to which she belongs). To what extent can she be her own person—i.e., be ethically autonomous— in these circumstances? The same kinds of difficulties, it should be noted, can arise for public health and visiting nurses, school and industrial nurses, and nurses working in extended care facilities. In these settings, the agency or organization for which nurses work places similar limits on their practice as the hospital. In the following chapters different cases will illustrate this problem of ethical autonomy, which is so basic to the consideration of ethics in nursing and so difficult to resolve.

We conclude this section with two important reminders about the notion of autonomy. First, autonomy does not mean unconditional freedom that would allow us to will or do anything. We are all aware of the formative influence of genes, culture, and social environment. Long before we were able to think for ourselves, each of us was provided with a set of emotions, beliefs, desires, principles, and so on. Nonetheless, how we use our natural, cultural, and social endowments in responding to the environment is, in varying degrees, up to us. As Gerald Dworkin has put it: "If the autonomous man cannot adopt his motivations *de novo*, he can still judge them after the fact. The autonomous individual is able to step back and formulate an attitude towards the factors that influence his behavior."[12] Autonomy, therefore, is compatible with a view of the world that includes a great deal of causal determination and constraints on our behavior.

Second, ethical autonomy involves thinking *for* oneself, not *of* oneself or *by* oneself. To think of oneself identifies the object and not the manner of one's thinking. Thinking by oneself, like "thinking for oneself," does designate a manner of thinking, but in ethics this manner of thinking is unlikely to yield the best results. Given the unrestricted frame of reference and complexity of ethical inquiry, thinking *for* oneself is usually more successful if it includes at least some thinking *with* others who can call one's attention to relevant considerations that one might otherwise have overlooked or misunderstood. This is why discussion with people of various relevant backgrounds is vital to sound ethical inquiry. Thus, we may conclude, being one's own person or ethically autonomous implies neither selfishness nor isolation. One may perfectly well think *for* oneself and still think *about* and *with* others.[13]

Notes

1. This case has been adapted from one examined in Roland R. Yarling, "Ethical Analysis of a Nursing Problem: The Scope of Nursing Practice in Disclosing the Truth to Terminal Patients," *Supervisor Nurse*, Part I (May, 1978), p. 40. For a detailed analysis of this case that applies many of the points made in this chapter, see the remainder of this article as well as Part II (June, 1978).
2. "Talk of the Town," *The New Yorker* (July 3, 1978), p. 19.
3. *Encyclopedia of Bioethics,* Warren T. Reich, editor-in-chief, (New York: Free Press, 1978), Vol. 4, p. 1789. All subsequent references to the Code's Interpretive Statements may be found here.
4. Yarling, p. 49.
5. Raymond S. Duff and A. G. M. Campbell, "Moral and Ethical Dilemmas in the Special-Care Nursery," *New England Journal of Medicine*, 289 (October 25, 1973), pp. 890–94.
6. John Stuart Mill, *On Liberty* (New York: Liberal Arts Press, 1956), p. 45.
7. Sarah Dock, "The Relation of the Nurse to the Doctor and the Doctor to the Nurse," *American Journal of Nursing*, 17 (1917), p. 394. Cited in Marjorie J. Stenberg, "The Search for a Conceptual Framework as a Philosophic Basis for Nursing Ethics: An Examination of Code, Contract, Context, and Covenant," *Military Medicine*, 144 (January, 1979), p. 10.
8. Stenberg, p. 8.
9. C. K. Hofling et al., "An Experimental Study in Nurse-Physician Relationships," *Journal of Nervous and Mental Disease,* 143 (1966), pp. 171–80.
10. *Ibid.*, p. 176.
11. *Ibid.*, p. 177.
12. Gerald Dworkin, "Autonomy and Behavior Control," *Hastings Center Report*, 6 (February, 1976), p. 24.

13. For two accounts of the concept of and format for ethics rounds as a way of institutionalizing ethical inquiry for nurses in the clinical context, see Anne Davis, "Ethics Rounds with Intensive Care Nurses," *Nursing Clinics of North America,* 14 (March, 1979), pp. 45–55; and Kathleen A. Mahon and Sally J. Everson, "Moral Outrage—Nurses' Right or Responsibility: Ethics Rounds for Nurses," *Journal of Continuing Education in Nursing,* 10 (No. 3, 1979), pp. 4–7.

2

Unavoidable Topics in Ethical Theory

1. Introduction

Ethical inquiry in everyday life and in health care often proceeds without formal recourse to ethical theory. Questions may be clarified, distinctions drawn, arguments examined, and solutions found without appealing to theoretical considerations about the nature and justification of basic moral principles. Thus, the fact that two people have different foundations for their ethical views is sometimes irrelevant to the resolution of a particular problem.

Suppose, for example, a question arises over whether everything possible should be done to prolong the life of an elderly man in a nursing home. Suppose, too, that he has no known family and that the decision must be made by the staff. One person, *A*, might argue that the man should be treated because not to do so would be to violate the duty to preserve and prolong life. Another person, *B*, might also argue that the man should be treated, but for different reasons. *B* may argue that the man is not in severe pain and that even though his mental capacities are significantly impaired, he seems to be reasonably content. Since it is *B*'s view that one ought, above all, to do what will maximize happiness, she believes that efforts to prolong the man's life should continue. So the issue in this case can be resolved despite the fact that *A* and *B* hold different basic principles and, perhaps, different conceptions of how they are known and justified.

Yet things do not always work out this way. Sometimes different positions on a particular ethical issue are a direct function of the parties' holding different ethical principles. In this event, the issue cannot be resolved without some discussion of the nature and justification of the ethical principles underlying the differing positions. Suppose, for example, that the facts in the case sketched above were altered so that the patient was experiencing unmitigable pain and distress. In this case, *B*, with her basic commitment to maximizing happiness, would have to revise her particular judgment and say that efforts to extend the man's life should no longer be as strenuous. The change in facts, however, would not be relevant to *A*, and her judgment that the patient's life should be prolonged would be the same. Here the resulting disagreement is rooted firmly in the difference between their basic principles. If they pursue the matter further, they will encounter questions about the nature and justification of ethical principles that have long been the subject of ethical theory.[1]

This chapter is a bare-bones introduction to three topics in theoretical ethics that cannot be avoided by anyone who seeks to develop systematic responses to ethical issues in nursing. First, we will make a brief survey of *basic* ethical principles and how they constrain or engender *secondary* principles. Then we will discuss knowledge in ethics and, in particular, the kinds of considerations that are relevant to determining whether one basic principle is more securely grounded than another. Finally, we will turn to the important question of the relationships and relative priority of ethical, legal, and religious considerations in a pluralistic society.

2. Basic ethical principles

Persons holding different ethical principles might well come to different conclusions about what ought to be done in the following case, which raises questions about how nursing care should be distributed when conditions are less than ideal.

2.1 Priorities: baby or parents?

Martha Schwartz, one of the most senior staff nurses in the neonatal intensive care unit, works only part time because of her own children. Baby Daniel Ingerman has coded, and Martha, with a recently graduated registered nurse at her side, is quickly and efficiently working with a house doctor to resuscitate him. It is clear, however, that the baby's chances of surviving this epsiode are extremely slim, and that even if he lives he will probably be severely handicapped both mentally and physically.

As she is about to help with a medication, Martha glances through the window at Elaine and Don Ingerman somberly watching the staff's frantic activity. At once she realizes that she should be in two places simultaneously. The parents need her; their child is dying. She has worked with the Ingermans during the past two critical days and believes she could be of help to them.

What should Martha Schwartz do in this case? Is it best to stay with the baby or go to the parents and let the other nurse assist in the emergency? Is the likelihood that the other nurse will be able to work less effectively than Martha with the doctor going to lessen the baby's already slim chances for survival? Is it fair to the young nurse, the doctor, or the baby to leave them in this situation? Or should Martha stay with the baby and send the new RN to be with the parents, people she's never met?

To see how basic ethical principles occupy a central role in ethical inquiry, consider the following excerpt from a fictional discussion of this case by three nurses.

Debbie: I definitely think that there is no problem here. There is only one thing that Martha can do. And that's to stay with the baby and do everything possible to help save its life. And the new RN, even though she may not be able to help the doctor, ought to stick around and learn how to be effective in such situations in the future.

Renee: Why do you say this?

Debbie: It's simple. The most basic duty of doctors and nurses is to save life. Sure it's important to communicate with parents and other family members when you can. But when you have to choose between that and honoring the duty to preserve and protect the patient's life, there's no choice. You go with the more basic duty, and no duty is more basic for us than preserving and prolonging the patient's life.

Ursula: Boy, nothing personal Debbie, but that kind of rigid, moralistic thinking really drives me up the wall. I mean how can you have so much confidence in an absolute rule like "Always preserve and protect life." I can think of lots of cases where the consequences of doing that would do nothing but make everybody more miserable. I really think we've got to get away from these old-fashioned, absolute "do's" and "don't's" and start being more realistic and flexible.

Debbie: Then what do you think Martha should do in this case?

Ursula: Well, I think she should do whatever would work out best for everyone. If she thinks that staying with the doctor would make more people happy, she should stay; and if going to talk with the parents would be best for everybody, then she should do that. You've got to be flexible, you know. You can't apply rigid rules without paying attention to the consequences.

Renee: Well, what do you think would have the best consequences *in this case?*

Ursula: Mmmm, that's hard to say. I think I need more facts and time to balance things out.

Debbie: Martha didn't have all that much time to "balance things out."

Ursula: O.K., assuming that the baby was going to die anyway or that even if he lived, his life would create enormous unhappiness for himself and everyone else, I think she should have gone to talk with the parents. This would relieve some of their anxiety and perhaps help them prepare for the grieving process. And the new RN would have an opportunity to get some valuable experience which will be useful when she is working on a code that would have better consequences than this one.

Debbie: You make it all sound so heartless and mechanical. What do you think Renee? Which of us is right?

Renee: I don't know. Frankly I don't think I can go along a hundred percent with either of you. For me the most important thing is to respect people's basic rights. I think lots of people have important rights in this case. The parents have a right to be supported and informed about what's going on. The baby has a right to life. The doctor has a right to the best available assistance. And the new RN has a right not to be abandoned in a situation in which she is over her head. The main problem in this case is that you can't satisfy all of these rights. So I guess you start with the most basic, which is, of course, the baby's right to life. And that means that Martha ought to stay with the baby.

Ursula: But I think your "right to life" is just as old-fashioned and rigid as Debbie's "duty to save life." As a matter of fact it's the same thing only inside out. And what good is a "right to life" if the consequences of honoring it makes everyone miserable, including the person whose life is saved?

Renee: I don't know, Ursula, except that I think that some things are right or wrong even if they don't have the best consequences or make everyone deliriously happy. And respecting people's basic right to life is one of these.

In this admittedly contrived discussion, each participant represents an ethical outlook that is anchored by a different sort of basic principle. Debbie's basic principles take the form of duties. Her framework is what we might call duty-based.[2] It holds that there are certain basic duties that must be performed *no matter what*. Although it does not deny the importance of maximizing happiness or respecting certain rights, these must always give way if they conflict with the performance of basic duties. Ursula, on the other hand, places the goal of maximizing the greatest general happiness at the base of her ethical framework. Everything in her framework is justified by appealing to maximizing happiness. Thus, if a conflict arises between acknowledging certain duties or rights on the one hand and maximizing happiness on the other, Ursula goes with the latter. Finally, Renee emphasizes the importance of people's basic rights. These rights occupy the same place in her framework as basic duties do in Debbie's. Although she does not deny the importance of human happiness, maximizing it is always to be constrained by respecting people's basic rights.

In the following discussion, four ethical frameworks will be examined more thoroughly. We begin with utilitarianism, or goal-based, theories and then turn to duty- and right-based theories which, despite their differences, are alike in holding that at least some acts are morally required apart from the extent to which they maximize happiness or any other overall goal. Then we conclude by discussing a framework that refuses to rank or weight basic goals, duties, and rights. First, however, it will be helpful to say a bit more about goals, duties, and rights.

Each of the four major types of ethical framework has three elements: overall goals, individual duties, and individual rights. (1) *Goals* are states of affairs, considered good in themselves, that ought, morally, to be maximized. Actions may therefore be evaluated by the extent to which they further or hinder the maximization of these overall goals. People for whom the maximization of such a goal overrides all other considerations in determining what, all things considered, ought to be done, are said to have a goal-based ethical framework. And when the goal is specified as something like the greatest general happiness or social welfare, the framework is that version of goal-based theory called *utilitarianism*. In the above dialogue Ursula can be classified as a utilitarian. (2) *Duties* apply to individuals. Within a particular framework, a person has a duty to carry out or refrain from a certain action if and only if the framework includes a rule or principle requiring or forbidding that type of action. If the framework includes some duties that ought to be performed even if certain overall goals recognized by the system would not be furthered (or even if they would be compromised), the framework is duty-based. One that includes a basic duty to save or preserve life, like that held by Debbie, is such a framework. (3) *Rights* are claims or entitlements possessed by individuals which require that others not interfere with their exercise of them or, in the case of "positive" as opposed to "negative rights,[3] that they provide the rightholder with something he or she wants or needs. As with duties, a person has a right to something within a particular framework if and only if it includes rules or principles specifying that right. If a framework includes some rights that must be respected regardless of how this will affect the pursuit of some of the framework's aggregate goals, it is right-based. Renee's position seems to be right-based.

What distinguishes the main types of ethical framework, then, is not their elements; for all include goals, duties, and rights. Rather, the critical feature is the way in which each framework *orders* these elements. Whether, in cases of moral conflict, certain goals, duties, or rights are always *basic*, as opposed to *derivative* or *subordinate*, is the crucial question in determining the structure of an ethical framework.

A. Utilitarian theories

Utilitarianism, in all of its forms, holds that the rightness or wrongness of an act is always a function of the extent to which its being performed or omitted will contribute to the goal of maximizing the overall good, which is construed variously as the total or average happiness or welfare. The application of the utilitarian principle may be direct (as in the "act-utilitarianism" of Jeremy Bentham and J. J. C. Smart) or indirect (as in the "rule-utilitarianism" of Richard Brandt),[4] but it remains the supreme principle of morality, the court of ultimate appeal on every moral issue.

Of course, utilitarians still talk about rights and duties, but these are always derived from the utilitarian principle. They have no independent standing. If, for example, including a right to freedom of speech would increase the chances of maximizing the overall goal, then this right would be included in the utilitarian's framework. Its status, however, would depend on its continuing to contribute to the utilitarian goal. In his celebrated defense of individual liberty, John Stuart Mill argues that "the sole end for which mankind are warranted, individually and collectively, in interfering with the liberty of action of any of their members is self-protection."[5] He adds, however, that the right to individual liberty is not basic, but rather derived from the principle of utility:

It is proper to state that I forego any advantage which could be derived to my argument from the idea of abstract right as a thing independent of utility. I regard utility as the ultimate appeal on ethical questions, but it must be utility in the largest sense, grounded on the permanent interests of man as a progressive being.[6]

In his view, then, if there were ever a clash between the claims of utility (the basic principle) and the right to freedom of speech or action (the derived principle), it would be the latter that would give way. Utilitarians like Mill, however, have argued that such an occurrence, though not impossible, is highly improbable.

Utilitarians can, in the same way, include certain duties in their framework. The connection between the goal of maximizing utility and the existence of individual rights and duties could be represented in a goal-based framework as follows:

BASIC: 1. GOAL (e.g., Maximize happiness)

DERIVATIVE: 2. RIGHTS   2. DUTIES

For a utilitarian, then, both the rights of patients and the duties of nurses and physicians are determined by appeal to the utilitarian principle. Whenever there is a conflict between such a right or duty and utility, the right or duty loses its source of justification. One consequence of this view is that *in principle* the utilitarian has a solution to every moral dilemma. All such dilemmas, which are construed as conflicts among rights and duties, can, in principle, be resolved by a fresh appeal to the facts of the case and the principle of utility. Whichever course of action promises to yield the greatest net balance of utility is the one that ought (morally) to be pursued.

B. Duty-based theories

Duty-based theories take some particular duty or set of duties as fundamental. Examples of such theories are those based on a duty to obey God's will as expressed, say, in the Ten Commandments, Kantian theory (especially the first formulation of the categorical imperative: "Act only on that maxim that you can will to be a universal law"), and traditional medical morality rooted in the "do's" and "don't's" of the Hippocratic tradition (such as "Do no harm"). In taking some duties as basic, such theories place what have been called "side-constraints"[7] on goals like the maximization of happiness. Although maximizing happiness may be regarded as an important goal in such theories, there is a limit on the means that can justifiably be employed to attain it. In particular, one cannot justify the violation of basic duties by appeals to utility because such duties are founded independently of utility and occupy a more central place in the framework in question. Frameworks in which duties to save or preserve life are basic, for example, do not allow an appeal to maximizing the total or average happiness to justify doing less than one's best to save a particular life. In such frameworks, saving or preserving life is believed to be right in itself, regardless of the consequences in terms of the greatest happiness. When conflicting duties make it impossible to uphold each one, a person has to consider the relative stringencies of the duties—supposing that they can be so ranked—or, if they are equally stringent, fairness becomes the main criterion. In extreme circumstances, one must consider utility to make the decision. Triage as a method for allocating medical and nursing resources under battlefield and other catastrophic conditions may have to be justified in this way within a duty-based theory.

Once the basic duties in such a theory have been identified, certain rights can be derived from them. Kant, for example, held that telling a lie was always a violation of a basic duty; and from this he derived the right not to be told a lie. We might, therefore, represent the structure of duty-based theories as follows:

BASIC: 1. DUTIES
                                                      ↓
DERIVATIVE: 2. RIGHTS
                                                ～～～～～～～～～

SUBORDINATE: 3. Goals
                                                     ↗↘
DERIVATIVE: 4. Rights   4. Duties

Here certain basic duties give rise to certain rights. Then, provided that a person does not violate these duties and rights at levels 1 and 2 he or she pursues certain goals, such as the maximization of happiness, at level 3. The wavy line emphasizes that the goals at level 3 cannot rightfully be pursued by violating the duties and rights at levels 1 and 2, which function as moral side-constraints on the pursuit of the goals at level 3. Finally, from the goals at level 3, we can derive nonbasic rights and duties at level 4. It follows that any possible conflict between the duties and rights at levels 1 and 2 and the duties and rights at level 4 are to be resolved in favor of the former, which are more basic to the overall framework. For example, suppose a nurse has a level 4 duty to obtain a patient's consent to her participation in a study. The level 4 duty is justified by appeal to the level 3 (utilitarian) value of the information sought by the study. But what if the nurse cannot obtain the patient's consent without lying to her and thus violating her level 1 Kantian duty to be truthful? Since the duty to be truthful is more basic than the duty to obtain the consent, the former prevails and the patient does not partici-pate in the study.

C. Right-based theories

In many respects, a right-based theory is, just as Ursula pointed out to Renee, a duty-based theory "inside-out." Its structure is as follows:

BASIC: 1. RIGHTS
                                                      ↓
DERIVATIVE: 2. DUTIES
                                                ～～～～～～～～～

SUBORDINATE: 3. Goals

DERIVATIVE: 4. Rights   4. Duties

The main difference between this and a duty-based framework is that level 1 is made up of fundamental rights, which then allow for the derivation of certain corresponding duties at level 2. Examples of right-based frameworks include Thomas Paine's defense of the American Revolution, John Rawls' *A Theory of Justice*, and arguments in the context of health care that turn, ultimately, on treating or respecting "the patient as a person." A case can also be made that Kant's second formulation of the categorical imperative ("Act so as to treat all persons as ends-in-themselves and never as means only") also provides the foundation of a right-based framework.

What, then, is the difference between a duty-based and right-based framework? Although they are alike in putting the individual at the center and in denying that the rightness or wrongness of an action is solely a function of its contribution to some overall goal, they differ in the extent to which they presuppose a relatively homogeneous set of values. Like goal-based theories, duty-based frameworks require significant agreement about what sorts of things are good for people. It is difficult to obtain agreement on a specific set of fundamental duties owed to others without some fairly clear conception of what is good for them or in their interest. In taking the Hippocratic Oath, the physician states: "I will apply dietetic measures for the benefit of the sick according to my ability and judgment; I will keep them from harm and injustice." This assumes that the doctor and the patient will share a relatively stable set of values that will allow them to agree upon what counts as "benefit" and "harm." Societies that are characterized by a great deal of agreement on social, metaphysical, and religious beliefs may be said to provide the appropriate background conditions for a duty-based ethical framework.

Where such agreement cannot be presupposed, however—where the conception of the human condition and of human well-being is pluralistic rather than monistic—right-based frameworks may seem more plausible. For unlike duty-based frameworks, they are "concerned with the independence rather than the conformity of individual action. They presuppose and protect the value of individual thought and choice."[8] By placing the rightholder at the center, such frameworks emphasize the individual's discretion to exercise (waive or transfer) a right to do or receive something *as he or she sees fit* and in a way that flows *from his or her values and life plan.* The recent emphasis on informed consent and the patient's *right* to accept or refuse health care is based, in part, on respecting the individual patient's values and life-plan. In a pluralistic society like ours, nurses and doctors can no longer be as confident as they once may have been that they know what counts as a *benefit* or *harm* for someone else.

D. Intuitionist theories

There is, finally, a type of ethical theory that includes no prior ordering of basic social goals, duties, and rights. Instead, each of these elements is accorded the same prima facie basic status, and dilemmas or conflicts between them are resolved on a case-by-case basis by comparing the relative "weights" of the conflicting prima facie goals, duties, and rights. The structure of such a framework is as follows.

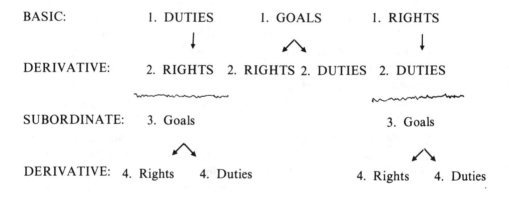

Someone who holds such a theory might respond to Case 2.1, "Baby or Parents," like this:

What makes this case problematic is that there is a conflict between Martha's basic duty to help save life and the basic right of the baby to the most skilled medical and nursing care on the one hand, and Martha's basic duty to respond to the parents' emotional needs on the other. But, all things considered, in this particular case the former outweigh (and not merely outnumber) the latter, so she ought to stay with the baby. But remember, things might be different if, for example, the choice were between staying with this baby, Daniel Ingerman, or leaving the new RN with him so she, Martha, could help out with another baby whose chances of survival and a normal life, if treated effectively, would be much better than Daniel's. In this case the basic goal of maximizing happiness may tip the balance toward responding to the baby whose chances of survival *with treatment* are significantly better than Daniel's.

If pressed as to how she "weighed" the conflicting rights, duties, and goals, the intuitionist would be unable to appeal to any more basic principles. For the conflict she is trying to resolve is *among* what she regards as a plurality of equally basic principles. Thus, her only recourse is to appeal to *intuition* or some sort of moral faculty, akin to sight as a visual faculty, that simply and directly informs her of what, on balance, is the right thing to do in this particular situation.

This completes our brief survey of the four ways of ordering the elements of an ethical framework. How are we to determine which of these four frameworks is best? To answer this question we must examine their relative strengths and weaknesses and the sense, if any, in which it is possible to know whether one framework is more firmly grounded than another.

3. Knowledge in ethics

The decision to adopt one or another basic ethical framework is extremely difficult because each has significant advantages and disadvantages. Utilitarianism, to take the prevailing goal-based theory, has a number of attractive features. It is highly sensitive to differences in factual circumstance and, apart from the principle of utility, has no rigid rules or principles that must be applied no matter what the consequences. As a single-principle theory it avoids the problem of conflicting basic rights or duties that can arise with other theories. For the utilitarian, then, there is in principle a solution to every moral dilemma—a way of making the best of every bad situation—by simply doing whatever is indicated by a correct application of the principle of utility. What could be more rational, one might think, than finding out which of the acts we might perform would, directly or indirectly, produce the greatest average or total happiness, and then doing it? It might seem, therefore, that to question this theory is, as Jeremy Bentham, the father of modern utilitarianism, put it, to "deal in sounds instead of sense, in caprice instead of reason, in darkness instead of light."[9]

Bentham's rhetoric notwithstanding, there are several problems with utilitarianism. First, there are significant *difficulties of application*. These include: (1) problems in defining *exactly what* each act is supposed to maximize; (2) problems in forecasting the consequences of possible courses of action quickly and accurately enough to ground decisions on utilitarian considerations; and (3) problems in comparing the happiness that a particular action will bring about in one person with the unhappiness it will bring about in another. Second, even if these difficulties of application can be overcome, there are serious questions about the apparent *implications* of utilitarianism.

For example, it has been argued that the maximization of happiness may require the punishment of the innocent, the enslavement or silencing of certain minorities, or even widespread euthanasia of the elderly and unfit.[10] Such possibilities arise, it has been suggested, because as a theory based entirely on maximizing the overall good, utilitarianism is unable to account for the independent value of justice or individual rights.[11] Although utilitarians may respond by pointing out that acts like punishing the innocent would *in fact* be likely to decrease rather than increase the overall good, they cannot rule such acts out on principle.

Duty-based frameworks, which occupy a prominent place in the history of ethics, have a number of advantages and disadvantages. In medicine and nursing, they are reflected in the traditional emphasis on codes of ethics. Duty-based frameworks appear to give clear, specific direction and thus are easily taught and passed on from one generation to another. Another advantage of their law-like form is the way in which duty-based frameworks readily lend themselves to enforcement. An ethical framework in the form of a set of relatively clear, specific duties makes it easier to identify immoral behavior and reduces the extent to which ignorance or slow-wittedness excuses it. Finally, duty-based frameworks make the relationship between a person's actions and his character very clear: a good person is one who does his duty. The connection between the moral worth of a person and the rightness or wrongness of his acts and judgments is not nearly so clear in other ethical frameworks.

Nevertheless, duty-based theories are subject to a number of objections. The most fundamental is that it is difficult to determine the content and justification of the basic duties. Often duty-based frameworks are versions of "divine command" theory, which maintains that the basic duties have their source in the will or law of God. But this does not solve our problem; it simply relocates it. For how are we to know what God wills or commands? If there is a disagreement about God's will or law, how do we determine whose conception is correct? Moreover, even if one could find a reasonably satisfactory account of the content and justification of the basic duties, it is unclear that any fully developed framework could be both comprehensive and consistent. If the set of basic duties is comprehensive, it is likely, given the complexity of human affairs, that situations will arise in which they would conflict; hence they would be inconsistent. If, on the other hand, efforts were made to eliminate such inconsistencies, they would probably also eliminate certain duties as basic, so that consistency would be purchased at the price of comprehensiveness. In addition, utilitarians criticize duty-based theories as overly rigid or heartless because there will invariably be instances where fulfilling a basic duty would either cause or fail to prevent considerable pain and suffering. Finally, insofar as duty-based theories, like goal-based theories, presuppose a widely shared conception of what is good for people or in their interest, they seem less at home in the emerging world community or in pluralistic nations like the United States than in traditional societies or more homogeneous nations.

A preference for right-based theories over goal- and duty-based theories is usually grounded on their compatibility with divergent conceptions of what is good for people or in their interest as well as with divergent religious beliefs. By emphasizing the intrinsic value of individual thought and choice, a right-based theory fosters tolerance and liberty and allows various conceptions of the good life to flourish. Underlying this is a respect for the dignity and autonomy of each person or, as Kant put it, our status as "ends-in-ourselves." To the extent that we are all ends-in-ourselves or have the capacity for rational choice, each of us has a basic right not to be treated as merely a means to an end or overall goal. Thus, a right-based theory supports our intuitions about justice and the equal worth and dignity of each person. As John Rawls argues, "each person possesses an inviolability founded on justice that even the welfare of society as a whole cannot override."[12]

The first difficulty right-based theories encounter is the same that duty-based theories confront: How do we determine the content and source of the basic rights? The early right-based theories maintained that the basic rights have their source in the will or law of God. But an appeal to God can no more settle a controversy over the content and source of our basic rights than it can for basic duties. Second, problems arise in determining who possesses basic rights. If the capacity for rational choice confers such rights, it seems that not all human beings have them (e.g., infants, the severely retarded, the senile) while some animals do (e.g., chimpanzees with extensive sign-language vocabularies). But if such rights are assigned to all and only human beings, how can merely belonging to a particular biological species, regardless of one's moral nature or cognitive capacities, be a sufficient basis for possessing the rights? Third, as with basic duties, a comprehensive set of basic rights will probably lead to conflicts when applied and hence be inconsistent. One possible solution, of course, is to rank basic human rights in order of relative stringency—but what nonutilitarian criteria are to be employed in doing this? Fourth, it is argued that at times respecting one person's basic right will require others to undergo an enormous loss of human happiness. As a reductio ad absurdum, it has been said that a right-based theory may require that "justice be done though the heavens fall and the masses perish."[13] Finally, by placing so much emphasis on individuality and independent choice, it is argued that a right-based theory makes it extremely difficult to preserve or develop a system of shared values and the valuable sense of community and belonging that goes with it.

Intuitionism attempts to preserve the most attractive features of the other frameworks by granting certain goals, duties, and rights a prominent place among its basic principles. In situations where these principles give conflicting guidance, persons can appeal to their moral intuition to determine which, all things considered, is overriding. With this flexibility built in, the intuitionist will never be forced into absurdity by prior commitment to a goal, duty, or right as more basic in every situation than any of the others. She will never have to sacrifice the right to life for a modest increase in overall happiness or pass up the opportunity to obtain a very large increase in happiness in order to honor a comparatively inconsequential basic duty or right.

Although in many ways a plausible and attractive framework, intuitionism raises a number of difficulties. First, insofar as it takes some goals, duties, and rights as basic, intuitionism encounters difficulties like those that attend goal-, duty-, and right-based frameworks. There will be problems in applying goal-based directives and problems in determining the content and justification of basic duties and rights. Moreover, a moment's reflection reveals that intuitionism's flexibility comes at a heavy price: it provides no criteria for resolving conflicts of intuitions. This limitation may not be very noticeable in everyday situations in a homogeneous, close-knit society where new circumstances are few and people's intuitions, because of their similar upbringings and the slow pace of social change, generally coincide. But the limitation becomes apparent in a context like that of modern health care in a pluralistic society. Issues in this context are in many ways unprecedented. They arise from recent advances in medical knowledge and technology and against the backdrop of social, cultural and legal change. Moral intuition, for example, cannot take us very far in resolving disagreements over the use of life-sustaining technology in an era of increasingly restricted medical resources. Since our "intuitions" largely derive from lessons learned as children, they are not easily applied to this issue, especially when a solution requires that a large number of people—patients, nurses, social workers, physicians, etc.—agree.[14]

This concludes our brief survey of the relative strengths and weaknesses of the four main types of ethical frameworks. The question now is whether we can know that one is better than the others, and if so, how. This important question about the nature and justification of ethical knowledge has been a matter of philosophical controversy for hundreds of years. Though we cannot even begin to address it adequately here, we believe that some version of what John Rawls has called the "method of wide reflective equilibrium" provides the best way to compare and evaluate ethical frameworks.[15]

Briefly, this method tests ethical theories by comparing the extent to which they produce coherence among three sets of beliefs: (1) our most secure moral judgments in individual cases (e.g., that it would be wrong to torture a child); (2) our moral principles ordered in a goal-based, duty-based, right-based, or intuitionist framework; and (3) a set of well-grounded background theories about such things as the nature of persons and the extent of human autonomy. To the extent that one or another ethical theory—represented mainly by the ordered set of principles that make up the second set of beliefs—satisfies the requirements of reflective equilibrium better than the others, it is, for the time being, the most adequate theory. The three sets of beliefs are said to be in "equilibrium" because they cohere; that is, they are mutually supportive, providing both clear justification for our most secure moral judgments and systematic approaches to problems where our intuitive responses are less secure or determinate. The equilibrium is said to be "reflective" because the preferred theory is based upon a continuous dialectical interplay between the three sets of beliefs and a willingness to re-open the comparison with other theories in the light of new evidence, arguments, or situations. As our analysis proceeds in this way, none of the three sets of beliefs enjoys privileged status. Elements of each may be modified, abandoned, or replaced in the interest of achieving a more consistent, comprehensive, and coherent equilibrium, or overall "fit," among them.

It follows that whatever theory seems to meet the conditions of reflective equilibrium better than the others does so only *provisionally.* As convinced as we may be of the superiority of one theory over the others, we should be prepared to re-open the question and re-examine our position. Our commitment should be a provisional one to what appears to us, *on reflection,* to be the best solution available.

We leave it to the reader, then, to partake in the lifelong personal and interpersonal task of determining which ethical theory, though falling short of perfection, comes out best under these conditions. Once we choose an ethical framework, we put it to use by: (1) trying to make our position on particular moral issues reflect it; (2) trying to refine the framework by working on its inconsistencies; and (3) trying to remain open to new or newly recognized implications, criticisms, and strengths of this framework that may prompt us to revise or replace it.

If what we have said about knowledge and justification in ethics is correct, there are two important consequences for ethical dilemmas in health care.

First, if all parties to a controversy rooted in disagreement over basic ethical principles were to take a systematic approach to knowledge and justification in ethics, they would be more likely to arrive at a resolution. As K. Danner Clouser has observed:

We generally quit the discussion of values long before we have exhausted meaningful argument. We are too quick to say, "You have your values and I have mine." Further discussion can elicit much more agreement either by pursuing the *consistency* of the value in question with other values that you hold or in "unpacking" the conceptual and empirical criteria underlying the value in question. Persistent pursuit of each other's values with "why" questions will elicit a lot of hidden assumptions and reasoning, and consequently more agreement than we would initially expect."[16]

Second, even where agreement is not reached, an extended, mutually respectful, reflective discussion will usually convince the parties that those holding opposing views are not thoughtless, callous, or otherwise "defective" from a moral standpoint. As a result, not only will lingering acrimony be limited, but the parties may also come to realize that, as thoughtful persons struggling with the complexities involved in justifying an ethical position, there is more that joins than divides them.

4. Ethics, law, and religion

Legal and religious considerations often play a prominent role in discussions of ethical issues. But to what extent and in what manner are law and religion relevant to the resolution of moral dilemmas in nursing? We may begin our brief inquiry into this difficult question by addressing the legal and religious considerations raised by the following case:

2.2 Religious and legal considerations in conflict

Jean Lyons, employed by the county health department, provided community nursing services to a rural area, including the schools. While Jean was at the high school, Kathy Jorea, a 17-year-old junior student, told her that she was pregnant but that she knew her parents, especially her mother, would never "get over it" if they found out. A friend had told her about someone who had had an abortion in a nearby city. Kathy believed that she must have an abortion, and she needed information about costs, the time it would take, and where to go.

Jean was strongly opposed to abortion on religious grounds. Appealing to the edicts of her church, she held that abortion was tantamount to murder, and she had become an active member of a "Right to Life" group shortly after the Supreme Court's Roe v. Wade decision (1973) had invalidated her state's legal prohibition on abortion. Over the past few years she had continued to support groups working toward a constitutional amendment prohibiting abortion. The thought of Kathy, healthy and obviously intelligent, destroying her baby, angered and frustrated Jean. The thought also crossed her mind that the county had few public health nurses and, since she alone covered Kathy's township, no other professional nurse was readily available to help Kathy.

In deciding how to respond to Kathy's request for information, how much weight should Jean give to her religiously based belief that abortion is as grave a moral wrong as murder? And to what extent does the fact that Kathy's abortion would, at present, be legal bear on her decision?

Let us begin by briefly examining the complex relationship between law and morality. The first thing to note is that although legal and moral prohibitions often coincide, certain acts may be morally, but not legally justified, and vice versa. In Chapter 1, for example, we assumed that a man taking his pregnant wife, whose labor has begun, to the hospital in the early hours of the morning is justified in cautiously driving through red lights. What he is morally obligated to do is nonetheless illegal. The circumstances may *excuse* him for violating the law, but they *do not suspend* the law. Similarly, abolitionists who violated the fugitive slave laws and civil disobedients, like Martin Luther King and his supporters, who violated certain laws as a last resort in protesting institutionalized racism, broke laws but did not act immorally. On the contrary, one may plausibly argue that what was immoral were laws that supported racism. In this case one would be saying that certain acts, though legally justified, are not morally justified.

The fact that we can identify acts that are morally justified but not legal, and vice versa, is not simply an indication of a remediable imperfection in our present legal framework. There will always be acts that are morally permissible or obligatory, but not legal, and vice versa. The former will occur because the completely unrestricted framework of ethical inquiry always allows for the possibility of new or unanticipated considerations overriding the prima facie moral obligation to obey the law. And the latter will always be with us because certain immoral acts (such as one person's falsely promising another to undertake long-term commitments solely to manipulate his or her consent to sexual relations) cannot be made illegal without resulting in either costly additions to the police force and unacceptable incursions on our liberty and privacy or an erosion of respect for the law in general. A simple appeal to an act's legal standing, therefore, is never a sufficient response to questions of ethical justification. And although a strong case can be made to show that in a reasonably just society individuals have a prima facie obligation to obey the law, it can be overriden in fulfilling a more stringent moral obligation.

How does all this bear on Jean Lyons' problem in "Religious and Legal Considerations in Conflict"? First, Jean might correctly argue that the legality of abortion (since 1973) is no more sufficient to show that it is morally justified than its illegality (before 1973) was sufficient to show that it was not morally justified. It is still possible, she might maintain, that abortion is morally wrong, even though legal, just as slavery in this country was morally wrong even when it was legal. So, *if* (and only if) Jean can provide strong reasons to show that abortion is tantamount to murder and hence morally wrong, regardless of present legal opinion, she may not only try to dissuade Kathy from seeking an abortion but also refuse to help her, withholding relevant information and possibly even notifying Kathy's parents of her predicament and intentions. Of course, this would include a refusal to provide certain legal nursing services and a breach of confidentiality—a serious violation of most codes of nursing ethics. Therefore, Jean's case for the immorality of abortion *must be extremely strong* if it is to justify such drastic measures.

Jean, we are told, is strongly opposed to abortion on religious grounds. Now, to what extent can arguments resting on religious belief be used to justify judgments about conduct in ethical dilemmas?

It is widely held that all ethical decisions are ultimately grounded upon, and inseparable from, some set of religious beliefs. If this is correct, people in a religiously pluralistic society will be unable to develop a systematic framework for resolving basic ethical disagreements. Ethical differences will be regarded as a function of religious differences and ethical reasoning and discussion will be interpreted as an attempt at religious conversion.

But what does it mean to say that ethical decisions are ultimately grounded upon, and inseparable from, religious belief? For some this may mean simply that our ethical principles are *historically* rooted in one or another religious tradition. Even if this is true, however, it does not follow that the principles cannot be justified on their own terms, quite apart from the tradition from which they developed. We do not, for example, say that the validity of modern chemistry depends on the validity of renaissance alchemy, even though the former had its origins in the latter; nor does the fact that astrology was the mother of modern astronomy imply that controversies arising in the latter cannot be resolved without appeal to the former. Similarly, even if there is a historical connection between religion and basic ethical principles, we cannot conclude that the validity of an ethical principle depends upon the validity of the religious tradition from which it emerged.

But when people claim that ethics is based on religion, they may also mean that religion alone can provide the ultimate justification of our most basic ethical principles. Many believe that an ethical principle is correct only if it has been issued by God. If this is true, a secular ethical framework will have no foundation, and basic ethical differences will be beyond the reach of reasoning and empirical evidence.

Nonetheless, we think that secular considerations offer at least as much support for basic ethical principles as religious considerations and that questions of public policy in a pluralistic society can be resolved only by appeal to secular arguments. In the previous section we suggested that the method of reflective equilibrium provides the most plausible approach to justifying ethical principles. Whatever cognitive difficulties attach to this method, they are no greater than the cognitive difficulties raised by the notion of God, or any other purely religious authority, as the ultimate source of ethical justification. Moreover, the striking similarity among the basic ethical principles held by people of widely diverse religious convictions is difficult to explain if ethical principles can be justified *only* within the context of religion. According to P. H. Nowell-Smith, this similarity

can be explained only on the hypothesis that when men think morally they think as they do when they think technologically—that is, rationally and on the basis of experience. The human needs that morality serves, nonaggression and cooperation, are everywhere the same; and it is not surprising that intelligent beings, reflecting on their own experience, have evolved broadly similar codes for meeting them.[17]

Thus, although people may attribute certain principles like the Golden Rule to religious authority, it is likely that insofar as these principles are widely accepted and presumed to be binding on believers and nonbelievers alike, they are also grounded on reason and empirical evidence.[18]

Our reasons for suggesting that questions of public policy be discussed in secular terms are mainly pragmatic. Agreement on basic policy in religiously heterogeneous societies like ours is possible only if the reasons for accepting such policies are independent of any particular religious doctrine. For example, patients and health professionals of various religious persuasions, as well as agnostics and atheists, will be able to reach agreement on recurring ethical issues in health care only if they can appeal to secular principles. Therefore, to the extent that it is important for people of differing religious convictions to adopt common basic policies, it is important that they support their views with secular arguments, even if their views had their origin in, and can also be supported by, religious arguments.

To suggest that basic ethical principles can be justified by secular considerations is not, however, to imply that people's religious beliefs, principles, and practices are irrelevant to the *content* of these principles. On the contrary, they are of central importance. To the degree that religious beliefs form a part of one's identity as a person, respecting the exercise of these beliefs is part of respecting the individual *as a person*. If a secular framework is to be acceptable to people of various religions, therefore, it should allow considerable freedom of religious observance and practice. In the context of health care, this will require that health professionals respect the importance of their clients' religious beliefs when these have bearing on decisions about their care. Thus, for example, religious holidays, dietary restrictions, and attitudes toward contraception, sterilization, autopsy, etc., will often be important in determining a client's course of treatment. Similarly, clients and various health care organizations and agencies must, where possible, respect the religious beliefs of various health professionals.

We may now apply this brief analysis of the relationship between ethics and religion to Jean Lyons' dilemma in "Religious and Legal Considerations in Conflict." The first thing to note is that Jean's opposition to abortion is based on her identification with particular religious ideals. This means that others, in their interactions with Jean, must, if they are to respect her, respect her personal views on abortion. But unless Jean can also provide strong, nonreligious arguments in support of her opposition to abortion, her personal, religiously grounded opposition is not sufficient to override her prima facie obligations to provide legal nursing services and to preserve the client's right to privacy. For if Jean's views are grounded in nothing more than religious teachings or conviction, any attempt to dissuade Kathy from seeking an abortion (assuming that Kathy does not share Jean's religious beliefs) would amount to an imposition of the nurse's religious beliefs on the client. And although people may try to convert others to their religious beliefs, the nurse-client encounter is certainly not the proper place for it.

There are reasonably strong, nonreligious arguments to show that abortion is a serious moral wrong.[19] The problem is, however, that there appear to be equally strong, nonreligious arguments showing that abortion is not a serious moral wrong and that it is, therefore, unjustifiable to prevent a woman who wants an abortion from obtaining one.[20] Thus, even if Jean's opposition to abortion were based on secular considerations, we may hope that attempts to anticipate and respond to objections to her position would have revealed to her that decent, thoughtful people—people who are neither callous nor "moral pygmies"—can hold an opposing view. Since purely religiously based convictions are inadmissible, secular arguments are inconclusive, and abortion is not illegal, we would state our position by saying that Jean must not interfere with Kathy's efforts and probably ought to give her the information she wants. But if she can find someone else to provide this information, Jean may be able to "conscientiously refuse" to do so (see Chapter 4, Section 3), referring Kathy to the other source.

Notes

1. A third possibility, agreement on ethical principles but disagreement on particular judgments, might arise when, for example, two people holding that one ought, above all, to maximize happiness disagree on whether treating a patient would in fact increase or decrease overall happiness.

2. The characterization of theories as duty-based, goal-based, and right-based that follows is heavily indebted to an analysis in Ronald Dworkin's *Taking Rights Seriously* (Cambridge, Mass.: Harvard University Press, 1977), pp. 169–173.

3. Rights, like the right to liberty or privacy, which require that others not interfere or otherwise encumber the right-holder's conduct, are called "negative" rights. They are contrasted with "positive" rights, like the right to an education or health care, which require not only that the right-holder not be interfered with or encumbered, but also that he or she be provided with certain goods. Generally, the case for "negative" rights is easier to make than the case for "positive" rights.

4. "Direct" or "act" utilitarianism holds that the rightness or wrongness of an action is a function of the extent to which the act itself contributes to the maximization of the good. "Indirect" or "rule" utilitarianism holds that the rightness or wrongness of an action is a function of the extent to which everyone's acting in accord with a rule contributes to the maximization to the good. Thus, act utilitarianism is *direct* insofar as it requires a fresh application of the utilitarian principle to each particular act to determine its rightness or wrongness; rule utilitarianism is *indirect* insofar as it requires that one always act in accord with certain moral rules which are, themselves, justified by an appeal to the utilitarian principle.

5. John Stuart Mill, *On Liberty* (New York: Liberal Arts Press, 1956), p. 13.

6. *Ibid.*, p. 14.

7. That is, one's pursuit of various valuable goals is *constrained* by having to abide by certain fundamental duties (or rights). Side-constraints function in some ways like certain rules in, say, basketball, which define the permissible ways of scoring. Prohibitions against double-dribbling and walking with the ball serve as side-constraints on a team's goal of making a basket. See Robert Nozick, *Anarchy, State, and Utopia* (New York: Basic Books, 1974), pp. 28–35.

8. Dworkin, p. 172.

9. Jeremy Bentham, *An Introduction to the Principles of Morals and Legislation,* Chapter I, "Of the Principle of Utility," reprinted in Edwin A. Burtt, ed., *The English Philosophers from Bacon to Mill* (New York: Random House, 1939), p. 791.

10. For a powerful, disturbing argument along these lines, see Richard G. Henson, "Utilitarianism and the Wrongness of Killing," *Philosophical Review,* LXXX (July, 1971), pp. 320–337.

11. John Rawls, *A Theory of Justice* (Cambridge, Mass.: Harvard, 1971), p. 26f.

12. Rawls, p. 3.

13. See Joel Feinberg, "Rawls and Intuitionism," In Norman Daniels, ed., *Reading Rawls* (New York: Basic Books, 1975) pp. 108–124, especially pp. 108–116.

14. See R. M. Hare, *The Language of Morals* (Oxford: Oxford University Press, 1952), pp. 74–78.

15. Rawls, pp. 19–22, 46–53, 577–587. See also Norman Daniels, "Wide Reflective Equilibrium and Theory Acceptance in Ethics," *Journal of Philosophy* LXXVI (May 1979), pp. 256–282. Versions of this method can be traced, historically, at least as far as Aristotle, *Nicomachean Ethics,* 1094v, 12-1096a, 10, bk. I ch. 3–4.

16. K. Danner Clouser, "Medical Ethics: Some Uses, Abuses, and Limitations," *New England Journal of Medicine,* 293 (August 21, 1975), p. 387.

17. P. H. Nowell-Smith, "Religion and Morality," in Paul Edwards, ed., *Encyclopedia of Philosophy,* Vol. 7 (New York: Macmillan and Free Press, 1967), p. 153.

18. See, for example, Alan Donagon, *The Theory of Morality* (Chicago: University of Chicago Press, 1977), especially pp. 1–9, 57–66; and R. M. Hare, *Freedom and Reason* (Oxford: Oxford University Press, 1963), especially pp. 86–111, 157–85.

19. See, for example, John T. Noonan, Jr., "An Almost Absolute Value in History," in John T. Noonan, ed., *The Morality of Abortion: Legal and Historical Perspectives* (Cambridge, Mass.: Harvard University Press, 1970), pp. 51–59; and Baruch Brody, *Abortion and the Sanctity of Life* (Cambridge, Mass.: M.I.T. Press, 1975).

20. See, for example, Judith Jarvis Thomson, "A Defense of Abortion," *Philosophy and Public Affairs,* 1 (Fall, 1971), pp. 47–66; and Michael Tooley, "A Defense of Abortion and Infanticide," in Joel Feinberg, ed., *The Problem of Abortion* (Belmont, Calif.: Wadsworth, 1973), pp. 51–91. The Feinberg anthology is a valuable source for strong philosophical arguments on both sides of this very difficult issue.

3

Nurses and Clients

1. Introduction

Moral dilemmas arising from encounters between nurses and clients generally raise one or more of the following questions. First, under what circumstances, if any, and for what reasons, if any, may a nurse treat an adult client as if he or she were a child? In other words, how can what we will call "parentalism"[1] be justified? Second, under what circumstances, if any, and for what reasons, if any, is a nurse justified in deceiving a client? Modes of deception may range from nonverbal pretense to withholding relevant information to outright lying. Third, under what circumstances, if any, and for what reasons, if any, may a nurse divulge information that has been given in private under the assumption that it would be held in confidence? And, fourth, how does the nurse determine to whom she owes fundamental allegiance when she cannot satisfy all of the interests or claims of those whom she has some prima facie obligation to serve? For example, if a nurse is supposed to be responsive to the needs of an entire family, what does she do when she cannot serve one member's needs or claims without failing to respond to those of others?

Although for the purposes of analysis we will examine each of these four kinds of questions separately, individual cases will often raise more than one of them. For example, one of the most common forms of parentalism involves deceiving patients in one way or another so that they will consent to procedures that the doctor or nurse believes to be "in their best interest" or "for their own good." The following case raises not only questions of parentalism and deception, but also questions about who ought to be regarded as the principal subject of nursing care and concern.

3.1 A helpful lie?

Public health nurse Linda Stone first met Arlene Knox when she was referred to the county public health department by an emergency room nurse who was concerned that Arlene's bouts of intoxication might be harmful to her unborn child. Linda soon learned that Arlene had previously been addicted to heroin; but when her boyfriend threatened to leave her, she had stopped taking the drug. Shortly thereafter Arlene had become pregnant. Over a period of several months Arlene repeatedly told Linda that she was no longer drinking; but Linda, aware of Arlene's past need for drugs and suspicious that she had not actually stopped drinking, continually worked to educate her about the danger of alcohol to the baby.

After delivery, Arlene's doctor told her the baby had fetal alcohol syndrome. When Linda made a home visit a few days later, Arlene was still crying and distraught and asked Linda to reassure her that she had not harmed the baby, that he did not have fetal alcohol syndrome. Linda suggested they both look at him, and she was surprised by his good health and vigor. He had none of the obvious signs of the syndrome. She immediately began to suspect that the physician had lied to Arlene in an attempt to shock her into an awareness of the seriousness of her drinking. Linda did not contradict the doctor, but told Arlene to ask him again. She also calmed her by pointing out the baby's strengths and by reassuring her that she would help her learn ways to stimulate his development over the next year.

Later Linda phoned the physician and learned she was right in suspecting a ruse; any problem the baby might have from alcohol would probably be small. The doctor said he would tell Arlene the case was slight when he next saw her, but he had no intention of changing his story since it seemed to make her realize what could have happened and, as a result, seemed to have strengthened her resolve to stop drinking.

Linda knew that lying and shocking Arlene was no substitute for helping her deal with the problems underlying her drinking. However, Linda also thought that she should perhaps also lie to Arlene; she definitely did not want to see Arlene drink excessively during another pregnancy and damage a child. Telling the truth might lead Arlene to believe she had no worry about the amount of alcohol she could consume during another pregnancy. Linda thought that she would begin to help Arlene with some of her under-

lying problems whether or not she contradicted the physician's story. After
several days of deliberation, Linda finally decided to go along with the
deception since, she reasoned, it seemed to be in Arlene's best interest.[2]

Insofar as Linda seems ultimately to justify her complicity in deceiving
Arlene by appealing to what she believes to be Arlene's best interest, the
justification is parentalistic. But there may be nonparentalistic factors in
Linda's mind as well. If Linda's concern for the welfare of Arlene's baby and
the children resulting from possible future pregnancies was the principal
basis of her decision, the justification would no longer be parentalistic. She
would not be deceiving Arlene mainly for her own good but for that of her
future children. Here, of course, questions arise as to whom Linda owes
fundamental allegiance: Arlene, the new baby, or possible future babies?
Finally, the deception in this case, as in most others, does not involve a
straightforward decision to tell a bald lie. It is more a question of withholding the truth. Of course, the situation is complicated by the fact that the
deception was initiated by the physician, and a decision to unmask it could
be costly to Linda's working relationship with him.

This brief discussion indicates just how complex cases of this kind can
become. To attempt to analyze them, the rest of this chapter will be divided,
somewhat artificially, into sections on parentalism, deception, confidentiality, and conflicting claims from different clients. Complications from the
involvement of a physician will be deferred until the following chapter. The
reader is reminded again, however, that in everyday life these considerations
frequently overlap.

2. Parentalism

In its most general sense, parentalism means that an adult is being treated as
if he or she were a child by persons acting as if they had the authority and
concern of a parent.[3] Just as a parent may force an unwilling child to go to
bed at a certain hour or take bitter medicine, so too, it is argued, a nurse may
sometimes force an unwilling patient to get rest or receive treatment. Like
the parent, the nurse will claim to be acting *on the behalf,* although *not at the
behest,* of the patient; for, like the child, the patient is presumed unable to
appreciate the connection between the nurse's behavior and his or her own
welfare.[4]

Where a parent forces or manipulates a child into doing something for his
or her own good, the assumption is that the child lacks the capacity to
understand, endorse, and act in accord with the parent's benevolent aims.

When a child is, in fact, able to understand and appreciate the parent's reasoning, but nonetheless disagrees with it, parental force or manipulation may no longer be justified. Thus, it is one thing for a parent to force a four-year-old to brush his or her teeth; it is quite another for a parent to prevent a fourteen-year-old from going to any but "G"-rated movies. Parents are justified in coercing or manipulating children into doing things "for their own good" when: (1) it is reasonably clear that the result will be in the child's interests; (2) the child is unable to understand or resists rational appeals to the connection between the act in question and his or her own (long-term) interests; and (3) it is reasonable to assume that, in the absence of special "brainwashing" or indoctrination, the child will endorse or ratify the parents' behavior at a later date when he or she can understand and appreciate the parents' aims and reasoning. It is because forcing four-year-olds to brush their teeth clearly meets all of these conditions, while preventing fourteen-year-olds from going to any "PG" movies does not, that we are inclined to think the former more justifiable than the latter.

Insofar as parentalistic coercion or manipulation of an adult involves a refusal to accept at face value the choices, wishes, or action of an individual who is presumed to be autonomous and self-determining, it bears an even heavier burden of justification. Parentalistic behavior, regardless of benevolent motives or the magnitude of the benefit to be secured or the harm to be avoided, overrides the right of an adult to be treated as a person. To be a person, as the term is used here, is to regard oneself as having the ability and right to formulate various projects and make various commitments, and then to attempt to fulfill them. A human being is identified as a particular person by the values and life plan that guide his or her conduct. To respect another as a person, then, is to take full account of his or her values and life plan and to give them as much consideration in determining the effects of one's conduct as one wants given to one's own values and life plan. Conversely, to disregard or give only perfunctory consideration to the values and life plans of others is to show contempt for them as persons. It is to regard them as mere objects or things rather than one's equals as persons, *even if one's aim is to benefit them or protect them from harm*. In Kant's terms, it is to treat them as mere means to an end, and not as ends-in-themselves.[5] And nothing is more demeaning to a person, more damaging to self-respect, than to be so treated. To deal with a sick individual as a person, then, is to place his or her values and plans, as far as possible, in the center of the picture and to attempt to preserve his or her sense of capacity for reflective choice.[6]

Nonetheless, as the following case illustrates, there may be times when an adult's capacity for reflective choice is seriously impaired.

3.2 Parentalistic restraint

Sixty-seven-year-old Henry Young had suffered a stroke and was being kept under continual restraint in the hospital at the direction of Kirsten Bennett, the supervising nurse. A locking waistbelt was used, whether Mr. Young was in bed or in a chair. The belt was of a "humane" design, permitting him as much freedom as possible while assuring that he could not fall out of the bed or chair.

Mr. Young had had a fall earlier in this hospital stay, having attempted to walk while unattended. He was only slightly injured in this episode, but because of the possibility of serious injury that such a fall presents, Kirsten required him to be restrained in the waistbelt whenever he was left unattended, even for a very short period. Mr. Young vigorously protested that he was being deprived of his dignity, that he felt as if he were in prison, that he was afraid of being unable to escape in the event of a fire, and that he was perfectly competent to be left free and responsible for his own safety. In response, Kirsten repeatedly told him that the restraint was a "standard procedure" for patients in his condition and that he had no choice in the matter as long as he remained in the hospital and his condition remained unchanged.

Underlying her decision was the fact that, as is not uncommon in such cases, Mr. Young's mental capacities seemed to swing back and forth so that sometimes he was undoubtedly competent to move about at liberty, but at other times he became confused and lost some degree of motor control. It had, in fact, been during such a confused period that he had suffered his earlier fall. Another important consideration was the fact that the nursing staff did not have time to keep continual watch over him. Thus, as Kirsten explained to Mr. Young's family, the restraint was "for his own good" even though contrary to his wishes. All things considered, she maintained, it was best for him to be kept in the waistbelt, even during periods of mental clarity, in order to insure that he would not, when unattended, lapse into mental confusion and seriously hurt himself. Mr. Young's family agreed with the supervising nurse and fully supported her decision.[7]

If we assume that Kirsten's appeal to Mr. Young's best interests is not a rationalization for a more basic concern with the hospital's legal liability, the convenience of the nursing staff, or an authoritarian desire to exercise complete control over all patients, her reasons for keeping him in restraints are purely parentalistic. She believes that Mr. Young's capacity to decide for himself on this question has been seriously impaired and that because he runs a significant risk of harm from being left unrestrained while unattended, he must, for his own good, be kept in the waistbelt even if he resists and protests. The question now is whether this parentalistic intervention is justifiable.

Parentalistic behavior requires justification because it refuses to accept at face value the choices, wishes, or actions of an individual who is presumed to be autonomous and self-determining. Thus, in justifying a particular parentalistic intervention, one must show that the presumption of autonomy or self-determination no longer holds—that the choices, wishes, or actions of the individual are not genuinely autonomous or authentically self-determined.[8] Even John Stuart Mill, whose defense of individual liberty is often considered to be antiparentalistic in the extreme,[9] allowed that we may interfere with a person's acting on his or her expressed desires when we can be certain that they are not his actual desires.

If either a public officer or anyone else saw a person attempting to cross a bridge which had been ascertained to be unsafe, and there were not time to warn him of this danger, they might seize him and turn him back without any real infringement of his liberty; *for liberty consists of doing what one desires, and he does not desire to fall into the river.*[10]

Similarly, we might conclude that Mr. Young does not desire to injure himself while walking around unattended. Thus, insofar as he is prevented from doing so, the nursing staff no more violates his right as a person to do what he (genuinely) wants to do than the intervener in Mill's example violates the rights of the person crossing the bridge.

In both Mill's example and the case of Mr. Young, the defense of the intervention rests on two conditions: (1) the ignorance or impaired capacity for rational reflection of the agent; and (2) the magnitude and probability of harm that would result without parentalistic intervention. Although some would argue that only the first of these conditions is *necessary* to justify parentalistic interference, and others would maintain that the second is by itself *sufficient* to justify such interference, we believe that both are necessary.[11] If a person meets condition (1), but does not thereby run an increased risk of significant harm, one cannot say that the "lesser evil" (the deprivation of liberty or choice) is justified by appeal to the avoidance of a "greater evil" (harm to the person whose liberty or choice is restricted); hence, the intervention is not clearly in the person's best interests. And if a person meets condition (2), but is mentally competent and fully aware of the magnitude and probability of harm that may result from his or her action, interference cannot be justified on parentalistic grounds unless one is willing to say that people should not be free to drive racing cars, smoke cigarettes, or refuse certain forms of medical treatment.

Although a parent may be justified in making a child do things judged to *benefit* the child as well as to protect him or her from harm, we believe that generally a health professional can override an adult client's right to self-determination *only to prevent harm*. Although the difference between preventing harm and providing a benefit is not always clear, often it is both clear and useful. The main difference between the promotion of benefit and the prevention of harm, for our purposes, is that it is much easier to obtain agreement on what constitutes a harm than on what constitutes a benefit. People may, for example, differ widely about whether public funds should be used to promote the arts, athletics, ethnic festivals, libraries, or parks, but there is usually significant agreement among the same people that such funds should be used to prevent foreign invasions, crime, and disease. The latter are regarded as harms of great magnitude by most any set of values, while whether one or another of the former is regarded as a vital benefit will vary widely from one set of values to another. Thus, unless one has a more or less explicit prior consent for interventions conceived mainly as providing a benefit rather than preventing a harm, the *presumed* benefit (which may simply reduce to the imposition of one's own values on a vulnerable patient) cannot override the *certain* infringement of a person's right to self-determination.

Underlying this emphasis on harm as opposed to benefit is an assumption that parentalistic behavior is justifiable only if the subject of the intervention in some sense consents to it. For example, a parent's forcing the child to brush his or her teeth is justified, in part, by the reasonable assumption that the child at a later date when the parent's aims and reasoning can be understood and appreciated, will endorse or ratify the parent's behavior. As Gerald Dworkin puts it, "Parental paternalism may be thought of as a wager by the parent on the subsequent recognition of the wisdom of the restrictions. There is an emphasis on what could be called future-oriented consent—on what the child will come to welcome, rather than on what he does welcome."[12] Similarly, just as Mr. Young, the stroke victim in Case 3.2, does not want to injure himself, and the person about to walk over the bridge in Mill's example does not want to fall into the river, those who parentalistically interfere can reasonably assume that their interventions will later be ratified by the subjects of the interference.[13] Thus, we may now add a future consent condition to the two we have already provided for the justification of an act of parentalism. An act of parentalism will now be said to be justified if and only if:

1. The subject is, under the circumstances, irretrievably ignorant of relevant information, or his or her capacity for rational reflection is significantly impaired;
2. The subject is likely to be significantly harmed unless interfered with; and
3. It is reasonable to assume that the subject will, at a later time, with greater knowledge or the recovery of his or her capacity for rational reflection, ratify the decision to interfere by consenting to it.[14]

Let us now become more thoroughly acquainted with these conditions for justifiable parentalism by applying them to two more cases.

3.3 Convincing the patient

"The job of a primary nurse," in Debbie Rokken's words, "is to provide care to the patients; and that includes basic assessment, basic nursing care, bathing, and different kinds of nursing duties; also more sophisticated care, such as giving chemotherapy, blood components, IVs, and medications. If I personally cannot give the care directly, then I have an LPN or an orderly who will work along with me to see that the care gets done. I work the three to eleven shift, and another RN from the day shift is my associate. Between the two of us, we organize the care and provide it to the same group of patients." In the primary care system the primary nurse, being ultimately responsible for the patient's nursing needs, exercises considerable influence over the patient.[15]

Debbie and her associate cared for Mrs. Cotton, who was thought to have metastasis to the pelvic area and for whom a total pelvic examination was recommended. Both nurses agreed to help Mrs. Cotton decide about having surgery, which "might be radical." Mrs. Cotton was apprehensive about surgery, afraid of losing control with the anesthesia, and afraid that the procedure would be too radical. According to Debbie, Mrs. Cotton "had very little support from her husband or her children; no one talked about surgery, much less helped her decide whether or not to have it done." Debbie had seen two women recently "do very well with similar extremely radical procedures." She also thought that the other alternatives, no treatment at all or a less radical treatment, would lead to a much more rapid demise and certainly a lowered quality of life with dependence on narcotics for pain. Therefore, she attempted to convince Mrs. Cotton that such surgery might be a good idea. Debbie spent time talking about why Mrs. Cotton needed the surgery and what could happen as a result of her not having it. She spent time with Mrs. Cotton and carefully chose interpersonal relations skills that might enhance feelings of trust. She sat close to Mrs. Cotton, occasionally held her hand, and once put her arm around her shoulders to comfort her. After several days Mrs. Cotton decided to undergo the surgery.

Months later Debbie reconsidered her actions, not because of Mrs. Cotton, whose pelvic mass was not malignant, but because in her words, "After more experience I saw a lot of women not do so well, and suffer more from that kind of treatment. It certainly makes you ask yourself whether you're doing them a service or not." Debbie's parentalistic intervention in this case seems to meet none of the conditions we have suggested as necessary to justify such an intervention. It does not meet the first condition because there is no evidence that Mrs. Cotton's capacity for rational reflection is impaired (her fears seem to be those that most people would have about major surgery), and her ignorance of the risks of the procedure could be remedied simply by providing her with information. Debbie's intervention does not meet the second condition because, as she later learns, her belief that Mrs. Cotton is likely to be significantly harmed by not having the operation is based on insufficient evidence. Debbie's initial assessment of the risks and benefits of the surgery were based on a sample of only two cases. Finally, for the same reason, Debbie could not reasonably assume that Mrs. Cotton would later consent to her interference and hence ratify it; thus the third condition was not met. We may, therefore, conclude that Debbie's parentalistic intervention in this case was not justified.

The question of justified parentalism also arises in the following case.

3.4 Breaking the cigarette habit

Twenty-three-year-old Fred Winston had attempted suicide by shooting himself in the head. He was hospitalized with permanent brain damage, which left him largely helpless and his body deformed by muscular contractions. He required assistance for almost every activity. He was usually incontinent, though this was attributed more to a lack of concern than to physical incapacity. In addition, his speech was barely audible, and the combination of brain damage and emotional difficulties resulted in stammering, repetitious speech patterns.

Fred failed to eat well, and his primary pleasures seemed to be watching television and smoking cigarettes. After his initial period of hospitalization, those responsible for his nursing care decided to try to limit his smoking "for his own good." Thus, he was often falsely informed that his cigarettes were all gone, or that there were only one or two left and he ought to save them for later, or that no one was available to supervise him while he smoked (a safety requirement necessary because of his limited fine motor control). The nursing staff reasoned that since he did not appear to care about what was in his own best interest, they would have to take measures to limit his smoking even if he protested.

When he sensed what was happening, Fred protested as strongly as his limitations would allow. In response to the nurses' explanation that what they were doing was for his own good, he insisted that since there was little hope that his condition would improve, he was entitled to whatever gave him pleasure at the present moment. Given his condition, he maintained, smoking was "for his own good." But inasmuch as his physical debilities and difficulties with speech limited his capacity to resist or vociferously protest the nurses' behavior, their will prevailed.[16]

Before determining whether the nursing staff's conduct meets our three conditions for *justifiable* parentalism, we may want to ask whether their actions are, at bottom, parentalistically motivated. Parentalistic reasons for forcing or manipulating people to do certain things often function as rather high-minded rationalizations for conduct that is actually motivated by anger or a concern for one's own advantage or convenience. In such cases parentalistic reasoning, which we may characterize as primarily other-regarding, simply acts to conceal reasoning that is basically self-regarding, though we may be reluctant to admit this—even to ourselves. In the case before us, for example, it would not be surprising if the nursing staff's behavior were motivated by an underlying, unarticulated anger with Fred. After all, patients like Fred are not likely to make the nurse's already difficult job any easier. He requires a great deal of care and shows a lack of respect and consideration for the nurses by his apparently willful incontinence. His failure to eat well is also likely to frustrate the nurses and, like most people, they are probably threatened to some degree by Fred's self-destructive repudiation of society and all they hold dear, regardless of what drove him to attempt suicide. Thus, it is important in this case for the nursing staff to determine whether their conduct is actually, or only apparently, parentalistic.

Even if their plan to help Fred cut down on his smoking is intended for his own good, and not simply a rationalized expression of anger, it does not meet the conditions we have set out for justified parentalism. It does not meet the first condition because, as far as we can tell from the case description, Fred is neither ignorant of the dangers of smoking nor is his capacity to reason about his decision less impaired than that of other smokers. (It should be noted that other patients in the same part of the hospital were, subject to safety rules, allowed to smoke as they wished). The staff's parentalistic behavior fails to meet the second condition, not because cigarette smoking is not harmful, but rather because it has not been regarded by the society as a whole to be *so* harmful that adults, after being duly warned, are not free to decide for themselves whether the benefits outweigh the risks. Consistency demands, then, that we regard the probability and magnitude of harm to Fred from smoking at this point no greater than that to Fred before his hospitalization or to other people in or out of the hospital. Finally, the nurses cannot reasonably assume that Fred will, at some later date, ratify their decision by consenting to it. As he himself suggests, given his limitations, the pleasure derived from smoking has taken on a greater significance than it had before his hospitalization. As these limitations are apparently permanent, it is unlikely that he will ever be able to replace the pleasures of smoking with anything else.

If the nurses' conduct is not an instance of justified parentalism, it must be regarded as an attempt to take advantage of Fred's dependence and vulnerability to impose their values on him. Surely if he were strong enough to smoke without supervision or to protest vociferously, the nursing staff would be forced to change their treatment of Fred. Insofar as their force prevails, so too does their will. This, of course, is not the first time that professional dominance has violated the rights of patients to be treated as persons. But here as elsewhere, a precedent for the violation of someone's personhood ought never to be confused with an ethical justification for it.

3. Deception

Deception is a form of manipulation, and manipulation, like coercion and rational persuasion, is a way of inducing others to do what one wants them to do. Before the forms and possible justifications of deception in the context of nursing are directly examined, it will be useful to compare and contrast manipulation with coercion and rational persuasion as ways of inducing clients to comply with various medical and nursing directives.

Rational persuasion consists of appealing to another person's rational capacities in order to influence his or her behavior. Reasons and information are provided for or against various courses of action with a view toward changing the other person's beliefs or conduct in some specific way. Ideally, rational persuasion is conceived as a dialogue in which the persons attempting to do the persuading recognize that those to whom they direct their arguments are their equals as persons. As Lawrence Stern has pointed out,

"There is, in general, no point in reasoning unless the other person is capable of seeing reason, getting the point. If he can do that he can also correct *me* if I am mistaken. We are co-members of the rational community."[17] Thus, for a nurse to obtain a client's compliance with one or another directive or procedure by rational persuasion or client education is to recognize and respect his or her personhood. It is, for this reason, ethically preferable in this interpersonal context as well as others. Despite her professional status, then, the nurse must be prepared to engage in genuine dialogue with the client, which means that the client must be allowed the same opportunity to alter the nurse's views that the nurse has to alter the client's views.

Manipulation, on the other hand, puts a premium on the results of one's intervention and less emphasis on the means. It is a mode of altering another's beliefs or behavior by subverting or by-passing his or her rational capacities. As Stern indicates, manipulation includes "such things as deceit, the deliberate by-passing of conscious processes, and various conditioning techniques (real or science fiction) which place belief or action beyond rational criticism."[18] Etymologically, the terms "management," as in the phrase "patient management," and "manipulation" both have to do with *handling* things ("hand" is "mano" in Italian and Spanish and "main" in French). Raymond Williams, in his study of language and cultural transformation, has pointed out that "The word *manage* seems to have come into English directly from *mannegiare*, It.—to handle and especially to handle or train horses."[19] Horses are not handled or managed as if they were persons; one needn't pay attention to their capacity for rational reflection or personhood because they haven't any. To treat a person in the same manner bears a heavy burden of justification. Manipulation of persons with the aim of achieving a certain result places an overriding value on that result. The benefits of the result, in the view of the manipulator, are more important than the moral and emotional costs to the manipulated individuals from disregarding their personhood and treating them as if, say, they were horses. On the face of it, then, nurses should be reluctant to resort to manipulating their clients unless there are strong ethical grounds for doing so.

There is an interesting contrast between manipulation and *coercion*, understood here as one person's bending another to his or her will by force or the threat of harm. As Stern has pointed out:

Coercion is not dialogue. But in a sense it is closer to dialogue than is manipulation. Generally speaking, when successful, coercion achieves only unwilling compliance with the wishes of the person who uses it. There is no change of belief on the part of the coerced person; nor does he lose his capacity to do otherwise should opportunity offer. He gives in but is not convinced; and he remains an independent center of action. By contrast, manipulation brings about willing compliance or psychological incapacity to do otherwise. Coercion leaves open the possibility of dialogue; manipulation forecloses it.[20]

This suggests that coercing clients to comply with nursing directives or procedures, though needing justification and falling short of the ideal of compliance grounded on rational persuasion, is in some ways preferable to manipulating them.

Instances of rational persuasion, manipulation, and coercion can be found in the case studies we have already set out in this chapter. Linda Stone's initial response to Arlene Knox's drinking problem in Case 3.1 is an attempt to educate her about the danger of alcohol for her baby and thus rationally persuade her to stop her heavy drinking. Later, however, she also supports the doctor's decision to rely on manipulation in order to curb her drinking problem. In Case 3.2, Kirsten Bennett decides to use coercion to restrict Mr. Young's freedom of movement in the hospital. She might, however, have been able to take advantage of his lucid periods to persuade him rationally that, all things considered, being restrained in the waistbelt whenever unattended was in his best interest. Case 3.3 provides an interesting example of nondeceptive manipulation. Here Debbie Rokken uses interpersonal relations skills to manipulate Mrs. Cotton's consent to surgery. Debbie's approach to Mrs. Cotton in this instance may be no more in the subject's best interest than that of an automobile salesman to a prospective buyer. Finally, in Case 3.4 the nursing staff first tries to manipulate Fred Winston into cutting down on his smoking, and when this effort fails, they fall back on force or coercion.

Deception is the most common form of manipulation but, as Debbie's use of "interpersonal relations skills" in Case 3.3 illustrates, it is not the only form. The clearest, most widely recognized form of deception is lying. To lie is to intentionally say what one believes to be false with the aim of having others come to believe that it is true. There are, however, a number of ways to deceive people apart from lying.[21] One may, for example, deceive people simply by one's nonverbal behavior. Pretending to be busy when you want to avoid an inveterate bore or faking left before cutting right while playing basketball are just two of many examples of nonverbal deception.

Verbal deception can also take other forms. Saying something that deliberately creates a false impression but, because it is literally true, is not a bald lie is nonetheless an act of deception. An example from a widely used logic text[22] provides a particularly apt illustration of this distinction. One night aboard a certain ship the first mate got drunk. The captain was rightly very angry at this serious offense, and despite the mate's pleas for a second chance, entered into the ship's log, "The mate was drunk last night." Smarting and eager for revenge, the mate struck back the following day by (truthfully) writing in the log, "The captain was sober last night." Now this joke trades on the distinction between saying what is literally true on the one hand and conveying a true impression on the other. When the mate writes, "The captain was sober last night," what he says is literally true, but in the context it creates a false impression—namely, that the captain was drunk *every other night.* Thus, we must not allow a fastidious preoccupation with lying to blind us to the important distinction between saying what is literally true and conveying a true impression.

Other modes of verbal deception turn on negative as opposed to positive verbal acts, such as intentionally refraining or forbearing from doing something.[23] Negative acts of deception include refraining from correcting an existing mistaken belief or allowing someone to acquire a mistaken belief. Anthony Shaw, a pediatric surgeon, provides an example of the former in an account of an encounter he had with the father of a newborn infant with Down's syndrome and an operable esophageal atresia and tracheoesophageal fistula:

After explaining the nature of the surgery to the distraught father, I offered him the operative consent. His pen hesitated briefly above the form and then as he signed, he muttered, "I have no choice, do I?" He didn't seem to expect an answer and I gave him none."[24]

But as Shaw admits in the next paragraph, the father's consent was not truly informed. "The answer . . . should have been 'You *do* have a choice. You might want to consider not signing the operative consent at all.'"[25] By withholding this crucial bit of information, then, the surgeon had manipulated the father into signing the consent form in a manner that was no less deceptive than if he had employed a straightforward lie.

To summarize this brief account of the various forms of deception, we may say that deception is a form of manipulation that is aimed at controlling people's behavior by inculcating, or allowing them to retain, false beliefs. As a form of manipulation it subverts people's rational capacities and restricts their autonomy. Insofar as a person acts on the basis of false beliefs that have been deliberately conveyed or uncorrected by others, his or her freedom and dignity as a person have been compromised.

All of the standard types of ethical frameworks surveyed in Chapter 2 contain principles or strong presumptions against deception. Although the grounds will differ from one type of framework to another, the result is the same: deception requires justification, and the burden of proof rests on those who wish to initiate or maintain deceptive acts.

Most duty-based frameworks include some form of basic duty against lying or deception. St. Augustine's religiously grounded, duty-based view held that God forbade all lies and that those who lie do so at the risk of endangering their immortal souls:

But every liar says the opposite of what he thinks in his heart, with purpose to deceive. Now it is evident that speech was given to man, not that men might therewith deceive one another, but that one man might make known his thoughts to another. To use speech, then, for the purpose of deception, and not for its appointed end, is a sin. Nor are we to suppose that there is any lie that is not a sin, because it is sometimes possible, by telling a lie, to do service to another.[26]

Such absolute prohibitions have also been claimed to rest on reason alone. Kant, for example, maintained that in lying a person "throws away and, as it were, annihilates his dignity as a man."[27] For, insofar as liars betray or abandon reason and rationality as the proper mode of interaction among persons, they betray or abandon the source of their moral worth. "To be truthful (honest) in all declarations, therefore, is a sacred and absolutely commanding decree of reason, limited by no expediency."[28] Although neither Augustine nor Kant allows for exceptions to the duty to be truthful, other duty-based theories may build certain exceptions into the duty. Thus, for example, a duty-based framework could hold that one has a duty to be truthful except in those situations where deception is *essential* to preserve or protect life. In this case the burden of proof would be upon the would-be deceiver to show that in this instance deception is in fact essential to preserve or protect life.

Right-based ethical frameworks ground the presumption against deception on a person's right to autonomy or self-determination. Since deception, as a type of manipulation, subverts or by-passes one's capacity to exercise rational deliberation and choice, it undermines one's personhood. As Alan Donagan puts it, the duty to be truthful rests

simply on the fact that the respect due to another as a rational creature forbids misinforming him, not only for evil ends, but even for good ones. In duping another by lying to him, you deprive him of the opportunity of exercising his judgment on the best evidence available to him. It is true that the activities of a lying busybody may sometimes bring about a desirable result; but they do it by refusing to those whom they manipulate the respect due to them.[29]

It is important to note, however, that this sort of case for truthfulness leaves open the possibility of deceiving young children, those with severe mental retardation or impairment, and others with a significantly diminished capacity for rational deliberation and choice. But even when one is justified in deceiving such persons, one must consider their capacity or potential for rational deliberation.

It is widely held that goal-based frameworks like utilitarianism allow much more leeway for deception than either right- or duty-based frameworks. Indeed, we have echoed this bit of conventional wisdom in our use of examples in the two preceding chapters. But the issue is not so clear. Although on short-run utilitarian grounds it may appear that deception would produce a greater net balance of happiness than truthfulness in many cases, a more long-run utilitarian outlook may indicate otherwise. As Sissela Bok has emphasized, those who engage in deception

often fail to consider the many ways in which deception can spread and give rise to practices very damaging to human communities. These practices clearly do not affect only isolated individuals. The veneer of social trust is often thin. As lies spread—by imitation, or in retaliation, or to forestall suspected deception—trust is damaged. Yet trust is a social good to be protected just as much as the air we breathe or the water we drink. When it is damaged, the community as a whole suffers; and when it is destroyed, societies falter and collapse.[30]

Thus, insofar as the consequences of each act of deception may have a corrosive effect on the sort of trust that is necessary for the preservation of essential, but fragile, social bonds, there is a strong utilitarian presumption against deception.

Given this presumption against deception common to all standard ethical frameworks, it comes as something of a surprise to learn that codes of medical and nursing ethics have traditionally been mute on the subject of truthfulness. Bok points out that through the years, the oaths, codes, and writings of physicians have made little or no mention of being truthful.[31] Nor, for example, is a concern for truthfulness reflected in the International Council of Nurses Code for Nurses (Appendix A).

Whatever the reasons for this omission, the contemporary shift of emphasis in health care from the parentalistic dominance of professionals to the individual rights of clients is now beginning to change professional codes. The so-called Patient's Bill of Rights, approved by the American Hospital Association in 1973 (Appendix C), recognizes the patient's right to "complete current information concerning his diagnosis, treatment, and prognosis in terms that the patient can be reasonably expected to understand," and his or her right to "information necessary to give informed consent prior to the start of any procedure and/or treatment." Such information, the document continues, should include but not necessarily be limited to the specific procedure and/or treatment, the medically significant risks involved, and the probable duration of incapacitation. Where medically significant alternatives for care or treatment exist, or when the patient requests information concerning medical alternatives, the patient has the right to such information.

This emphasis on honestly informing the patient is echoed in the most recent version of the American Nurses' Association Code for Nurses in Interpretive Statement 1.1, Self-Determination of Clients. This shift to truthfulness places a clear burden of proof on any health professional who decides to engage in any form of deception.

Yet this burden of proof can sometimes be met. The question is: under what conditions and for what reasons is it permissible or obligatory to deceive a client? In what follows we will try, through a consideration of cases, to address this question.

3.5 Giving placebos

Sandra Seamans, staff nurse on a surgical unit, is caring for Mrs. Dorothy Langley, whose doctor has ordered placebos to wean her off Demerol injections that she has persistently requested since being hospitalized after a car accident. The day nurses have already given Mrs. Langley two injections of sterile water, each of which seemed to relieve her pain for several hours. Sandra does not want to give a placebo. She is worried about what she will say if Mrs. Langley should ask what medication she is giving. She has thought about warding off such questions with an "Oh, the same thing you got last time" to avoid lying; Sandra does not believe in lying to patients. Yet she acknowledges that, "You can't tell the patient it's a placebo because that ruins the whole effect. I know placebos are given to help the patient—to ease off medication and to allow evaluation of pain. But it is still going behind the patient's back and I don't feel comfortable with it."

Before determining under what conditions Sandra could be considered to be participating in a justifiable act of deception, let us briefly call attention to the way in which this case illustrates the distinction between telling the literal truth and conveying a true impression.

First, since the effectiveness of the placebo requires Mrs. Langley to believe that she is receiving biochemically active medication, she is deceived even if she is never actually told a lie. Second, even if Sandra should respond to a question from Mrs. Langley about her medication by saying what is literally true ("It's the same thing that you got earlier") she nonetheless conveys a false impression. Sandra would be compounding deception with self-deception if she were to believe that there is a significant ethical difference between saying "It's Demerol" and "It's the same thing you got last time."

We turn now to the question of justification. It is, in general, much more difficult to justify administering placebos than is commonly supposed. Too often, for example, the administration of placebos reinforces the patient's mistaken belief that there is a "pill for every ill." As a result, patients often fail to understand the inevitability of certain aches and discomforts, the limitations of medical understanding and techniques, the healing power of time, the importance to health of certain patterns of living, and so on.[32] In addition, the cavalier administration of placebos involves needless expense. But most important is the corrosive effect of placebos on the trust which is an essential element in the relationships between patients and health professionals. As Bok points out,

the practice of giving placebos is wasteful of a very precious good: the trust on which so much in the medical relationship depends. The trust of those patients who find out they have been duped is lost, sometimes irretrievably. They may then lose confidence in physicians and even in bona fide medication which they may need in the future.[33]

Finally, it is important to distinguish the placebo *effect* from the administration of placebos. The former is a way of characterizing healing that is attributable to the interaction between patient and professional, though not to any specific medication. The placebo effect adds greatly to the professional's effectiveness and requires no deception. It must be noted, however, that an indiscriminate reliance on placebos, which do require deception, will in the long run severely impair the capacity of nurses and physicians to take therapeutic advantage of the placebo effect.[34]

It follows, then, that placebos should be used with great reluctance and only when nondeceptive means to the desired end have been exhausted. For the sake of analysis we will assume that various nondeceptive attempts to reduce Mrs. Langley's dependence on Demerol have been eliminated on grounds other than convenience or expedience. Thus, we assume that Mrs. Langley has been unresponsive to attempts to educate her about the danger of addiction and to persuade her rationally to go without Demerol. Further, we assume that she is indeed running a significant risk of addiction, that in her present mental state further efforts at persuasion will be fruitless, and that her apprehension about the drug's being cut off will significantly magnify her pain and distress. If these assumptions do not hold, then we believe that the resort to placebo has been premature. But if they do hold, there is a fairly strong parentalistic justification for employing a placebo.

Recall the three conditions set out in Section 2 for justifiable parentalism. If, as we have assumed, Mrs. Langley has been unresponsive to education and rational persuasion about the dangers of addiction, we can infer that her capacity for rational reflection has been impaired (either by the drug or by her inordinate fear of the temporary pain and distress of being weaned from it); thus the first condition will have been met. The second condition will be met if significant harm is likely to result if she is not given the placebo; and it appears that it will. And the third condition will be satisfied because it is reasonable to assume that when Mrs. Langley is successfully weaned from the Demerol and informed about the way in which it was done, she will ratify or endorse the deception by retroactively consenting to it.

The following deception, although seemingly innocent, is much more difficult to justify.

3.6 "You won't feel a thing"

Amanda Adams and two other public health nurses offer an immunization clinic once each month in a conveniently located church. Amanda and her colleagues try to dispel children's fears of medical personnel by wearing pleasant, attractive clothing rather than white uniforms and by being friendly and cheerful.

One busy afternoon when the clinic was unusually crowded, David Winn, a five-year-old, was becoming apprehensive while waiting to get his rubella shot. When his turn came, David reluctantly walked with Amanda and his mother to an area behind a screen usually used to separate Sunday school classes. As Amanda picked up the syringe, David started to cry softly. Amanda noticed his distress and feared that he was building up to a long, loud scream that would upset those children who were still waiting. So, she smiled and reassuringly said, "Don't worry, you won't feel a thing." Then as quickly as she could she gave the injection. Although he did not cry out, David winced and emitted a little gasp as the needle entered his arm.

It is ironic that after trying to allay the children's fears through special attention to clothing and friendliness, Amanda's panicky lie to David is likely to compound his subsequent fear of doctors and nurses with mistrust. Trust is perhaps the most important element in the nurse-client relationship, and once lost it is exceedingly difficult to regain. If what David felt was not as bad as he had anticipated, it was nonetheless worse than Amanda said it would be. The next time a nurse attempts truthfully to mitigate his fears, it would not be surprising if his response were suspicious.

To conclude this brief discussion of deception in nursing, we want to emphasize that the presumption on behalf of being truthful does not imply that clients have an obligation to learn about their illness or treatment. Although people generally have a right to such information, they may, if they wish, choose not to exercise it. Just as a right to freedom of speech does not imply an obligation to speak, so too the right to be informed about one's illness and treatment does not imply an obligation to be so informed. Clients may indicate that they would rather not know all they are entitled to know.

3.7 Deciding how much to tell

The nurses on a particular medical unit always try to sit down and talk to patients before they begin their chemotherapy. Depending on the patient's ability to understand and accept information about the side effects of chemotherapy, the information they provide is more or less detailed.

In John Coughlin's case, the nurses felt that they had a responsibility to give more instruction than he had received from the doctor. However, Mr. Coughlin, a forty-nine-year-old carpenter, was extremely anxious about receiving chemotherapy at all. He tried to keep his mind and conversation on other things and would only say, half-joking, that he was sure that the chemotherapy was going to turn him into a "snivelling idiot."

After consulting with a colleague, Diane Fetterson, a staff nurse, decided that Mr. Coughlin did not want detailed information about certain side effects and possible complications. Therefore, before his chemotherapy began, Diane explained that he might become nauseated; he might lose some of his hair; he might not feel like eating; and he would need to drink many fluids. However, she did not tell him everything she might have told other patients. She withheld more detailed information that she thought would be needlessly distressing to Mr. Coughlin in his present state and which he, himself, had indirectly indicated that he did not want. As Diane put it, she was sure that he did not want to know all of the "gory side effects that could occur."

Although Diane withheld certain information, we would not characterize her conduct as deceptive. Insofar as we assume that Mr. Coughlin had chosen not to exercise his right to know more about the side effects of chemotherapy, Diane was under no obligation to tell him more. To have done so in this case would have been to confuse a right to be informed with an obligation to be informed.

As nurses and doctors rightfully move away from a norm of parentalistic deception, they must be careful not to embrace a norm of parentalistic honesty. If patients clearly indicate that they do not want to know more about their illness or treatment, it is not up to the health care profession to make stronger persons of them or to bring them up to some ideal of lucid awareness. Here, as elsewhere, genuine respect for persons requires sensitivity to genuine personal differences.

4. Confidentiality

An obligation to preserve the client's privacy and hold certain information in strict confidence has long been a part of nursing and medical ethics. As Point 2 of the American Nurses' Association Code for Nurses states: "The nurse safeguards the client's right to privacy by judiciously protecting information of a confidential nature." As with deception, each of the main types of ethical framework will include a strong presumption against disclosing information about a client that has been obtained under the supposition that it will be held in confidence.

Duty-based frameworks, which underlie most codes of nursing and medical ethics, will include a duty to protect information acquired within the clinical encounter. Right-based theories will emphasize the client's right to privacy and the confidential nature of communications and records pertaining to his or her care (see Points 6 and 7 of the Statement on a Patient's Bill of Rights, Appendix C). Goal-based theories like utilitarianism will base this presumption on the negative long-term effects of arbitrary disclosure of information given in confidence. Such a line of reasoning can be found in Interpretive Statement 2.3 of the ANA Code: "The nurse-client relationship is built on trust. This relationship could be destroyed and the client's welfare and reputation jeopardized by injudicious disclosure of information provided in confidence." After all, if clients were afraid that certain embarrassing or incriminating information about themselves would be arbitrarily or maliciously disseminated by health care professionals, they would be disinclined to share such information, often to the detriment of their health.

Nonetheless, as with deception, there are cases in which the presumption against disclosing information obtained in the clinical encounter can be overridden. Health care professionals are required by law to report cases of venereal disease, gunshot wounds, and child abuse even though they learn of them within the clinical encounter with its presumption of confidentiality. Reporting such information to government agencies, though not uncontroversial, is frequently defended because it is designed to protect the public interest. In addition, it can be argued that such acts of disclosure do not involve a breach of confidentiality because, insofar as the relevant laws are public and knowable in advance, the health care provider does not obtain the information in question under the supposition that it will be held in confidence. More troublesome, however, are ethical dilemmas about confidentiality that do not involve a prior suspension of the principle of confidentiality. Consider, for example, the following case.

3.8 "I don't want anybody to know"

Sandy Wilson, fourteen years old, had just completed a six-month check-up for a fractured ankle. The fracture had healed completely without complications, but her hemoglobin was in the low normal range. As a precautionary measure she was sent to Maria Garza, a nurse practitioner, for diet counseling. Before long Sandy confided that she thought she was pregnant and that she did not want anyone else to know, especially her mother. Upon brief questioning, it became evident to Maria that Sandy had no clear idea of what she was going to do about the suspected pregnancy. Before Maria could begin to help her think the situation through, however, Mrs. Wilson came in. Mrs. Wilson said that Sandy had been nauseated and very tired lately, and she asked Maria if she had any idea of what could be causing it. As Maria prepared to respond, Sandy remained silent and glared at her.[35]

Although there is a presumption that nurses should maintain confidence, there is also a presumption against deception. Maria's dilemma in this case is due to a conflict between these presumptions.

A decision to override the presumption against deception for the sake of confidentiality could be based upon the importance of maintaining trust in the nurse-client relationship. Maria is well aware that a young pregnant girl's trust in her, as a nurse, must be preserved. Moreover, since the law in their state does not require Maria to tell parents about a fourteen-year old's sexual activities, there is no legal ground for suspending confidentiality.

On the other hand, arguments can be made for truthfully answering Mrs. Wilson's questions. Although the presumption for maintaining confidentiality is strong, the ANA code states that information of a confidential nature must be judiciously, not absolutely, protected.

When knowledge gained in confidence is relevant or essential to others involved in planning or implementing the client's care, professional judgment is used in sharing it. Only information pertinent to a client's treatment and welfare is disclosed and only to those directly concerned with the client's care. The rights, well-being and safety of the individual client should be the determining factors in arriving at this decision. (Statement 2.1)

This statement provides a basis for arguing that "professional judgment" in this case dictates that the nurse should share information with the mother since it relates directly to Sandy's "well-being and safety." Teenage pregnancies pose a high risk to both mother and baby. If Sandy decides (or has already decided) not to have an abortion, obtaining good prenatal care is important and Sandy's mother may be instrumental in helping her get it. If Sandy does want an abortion, her mother could help her by arranging the abortion and, perhaps, by giving emotional support.

Another reason for being truthful with Mrs. Wilson is to refrain from reinforcing Sandy's avoidance of her problems. If Maria were to support Sandy's deception, she would undercut her own professional efforts to help Sandy develop effective ways of coping with difficult problems.

Given the limited information available to Maria, choosing between maintaining confidence and avoiding deception is very difficult. We hope that Maria would try to soften the dilemma by asking if Mrs. Wilson would leave the room for a short while so that she could talk to Sandy alone. Maria would then have time to assess Sandy's perception of family relationships. Maria could also indicate why she would like Sandy to release her from confidence so that Maria could deal more openly with Mrs. Wilson. If Sandy agreed, they could decide when and how best to tell Mrs. Wilson about the situation.

If Sandy does not release her, however, Maria would have to determine whether Mrs. Wilson's having knowledge of the suspected pregnancy would in any way jeopardize Sandy's well-being. If the knowledge would not place Sandy in jeopardy, either physically or psychologically, we believe that Maria has several reasons for telling Mrs. Wilson. First, Maria could justify breaking confidence on parentalistic grounds if: Sandy seems not to appreciate the situation or is unable to deal with it; the pregnancy puts her at risk; and in the future a good chance exists that she will look back and agree that involving her mother was the right course of action. Maria could also justify breaking confidence on the grounds that, if Sandy does not choose abortion, the unborn baby's claims to health care override Sandy's claims to confidentiality. Finally, Maria could justify breaking confidence on the grounds that Mrs. Wilson's rights as a parent override Sandy's right to secrecy. The mother's responsibility for her daughter requires that she be informed of current or potential problems. To do less would be to hinder her exercise of parental responsibility.

5. Conflicting claims

In Case 3.8 the nurse had to balance her obligations among three parties: the young girl, her mother, and her potential child. Whose needs or claims are to be given priority when a nurse cannot respond to all of those to whom she has a prima facie obligation? Consider, for example, the following case.

3.9 Who is the client?

Louise Russell, staff public health nurse serving the inner city, made a home visit to Mrs. Kathryn Simmons and her young baby. During the visit Kathryn told Louise that she thought she might be pregnant again. Not one to seek medical care until absolutely necessary, Kathryn hadn't planned to see her doctor. Louise immediately reminded Kathryn that her doctor had increased her epilepsy medication just after her baby's birth, and that she would probably need to get the prescription changed to safeguard the unborn baby's development. After a short discussion about the importance of checking her medication if she were pregnant, Kathryn phoned for a doctor's appointment. When Louise left Kathryn that day, she was pleased that Kathryn had assumed responsibility for herself and her unborn child rather than letting Louise take control and call the doctor for her.

A week later Louise wondered if Kathryn had actually seen the doctor. Although Kathryn had made the phone call in her presence, she was not convinced that she would follow through. She wondered if she should call Kathryn and check if she had, but she knew that Kathryn would immediately understand the unspoken message that Louise did not entirely trust her. Or, Louise thought, she could call the doctor and find out if Kathryn had kept the appointment, which would also be an admission that Louise did not trust her client. In the past Louise had struggled with the question of whether she trusted clients to act on information she gave them. But in this situation she had to consider the unborn baby, too. She didn't know how to balance her respect for Kathryn as a person against her responsibility as a nurse to protect the health of the unborn child.

Louise's dilemma is clearly drawn: if she treats Kathryn as a responsible adult, harm may come to the fetus; while if she intervenes on behalf of the fetus, she will not be treating Kathryn as a fully responsible adult. Although the case raises a number of different issues, our primary concern is this: whose interests, Kathryn's or the unborn child's, ought to be given priority when Louise cannot, on the face of it, satisfy both?

In cases like this we would suggest applying the principle that the client who runs the greatest risk of significant harm should be the primary concern. Thus, Louise should insure that Kathryn keeps her appointment because the risk of significant harm to the unborn baby if she does not keep it is higher than the risk of significant harm to Kathryn if she is upset by Louise's intervention. An important consideration in making this judgment is that it would be much easier for Louise to repair Kathryn's wounded self-esteem than it would be to reverse the harm that might befall the fetus in the event that Kathryn neglects to have her medication changed.

The principle we have appealed to does not imply either that Kathryn has no right to be regarded as a responsible adult or that a fetus's or child's rights always outweigh those of a parent or adult. First, both Kathryn and the unborn baby have a right to Louise's respect and concern. In this case, however, the fact that the unborn baby runs a greater risk of significant harm than Kathryn gives Louise strong grounds for overriding Kathryn's right. To say that Kathryn has a right that Louise has reluctantly overridden in the name of the unborn baby's more stringent right implies that Louise ought to do what she can to justify her act to Kathryn and indicate in other ways her respect for her as a person. Second, there may be occasions when the foregoing principle will indicate that it is a child's, and not an adult's, right to respect and concern that must be overridden. Thus, for example, if Louise makes a routine home visit to assess the development of a premature infant and discovers the mother with a badly infected cut on her leg requiring immediate treatment, her first concern should be with the mother.

Although we think it is fairly clear that Louise ought to insure that Kathryn has visited the doctor, it is not so clear whether she should do this by simply calling Kathryn or by calling the doctor. On the one hand, it may seem better to call the doctor. If the doctor indicates that Kathryn has kept the appointment, Kathryn may never learn of Louise's doubts; and the doctor's confirmation that Kathryn has kept the appointment is, perhaps, stronger evidence than Kathryn's saying that she has done so. On the other hand, making the initial call to the doctor shows less trust in Kathryn than calling her directly; and if she has in fact not visited the doctor and learns that Louise has been checking up on her "behind her back," the perceived insult and breach of trust will seem greater and the relationship between her and Louise will be more difficult to repair. We leave it to the reader to determine which of these alternatives is preferable and why. A more difficult case of competing client claims is the following:

3.10 Advocate for parents and children

As the community health nurse assigned to the city's northwest corner, Sharon Brinker believes that she is responsible to all the people on her case load. Recently, she was called into court to testify in a child abuse and neglect case involving Larry and Carolyn Trice and their three children, David, seven years, Linda, five; and Sandra, four. Sharon found it difficult to think in terms of individual clients because she usually looks at a family as a whole. Yet the court considers a child's welfare and safety separately from a parent's wishes for the family to remain together. One option before the court is to place the Trice children in a local institution that offers therapy to whole families; children are returned to parents who successfully participate in treatment programs. Other options require more lasting separation. The judge will base his decision in part on the recommendation of expert witnesses—doctors, nurses, psychologists, social workers, etc.

Sharon first met the Trices six months ago when David was unable to stay awake in school. She thinks she has made good progress with Carolyn in that she has gained her trust and good will. David has been doing better since Sharon suggested that Carolyn could leave food out for him to eat before school. But many problems remain, including some relating to David's asthma. Carolyn cannot or will not keep medical appointments for David, enforce rules for the children, or keep the children on any kind of a simple routine of meals or scheduled bedtimes. Larry, who works seasonally at pouring cement, usually takes little interest in the children's daily activities.

Recently, Linda has been caught stealing repeatedly from local stores on her way to and from kindergarten, with the result that Larry or Carolyn or both beat her badly enough to result in the court hearing. Sharon feels responsible for the children. She thinks that Linda especially needs her protection; if she steals again, she will probably be beaten. But Sharon also believes that the children need their parents. She thinks she must be the parents' advocate as well as the children's. She has built a positive relationship with Carolyn and thinks that, though she cannot meet all of Carolyn's many needs, Carolyn's trust in her as a professional and friend should be protected.

Sharon's problem is to determine what she could say to the court that would best preserve Carolyn's trust, protect the children, and preserve the integrity of the family.

Those, like Sharon, who consider the family or a similar social group as the unit of nursing or medical care occasionally find themselves in the following dilemma: If they do what appears best for the family as a whole, they may violate the rights or neglect basic needs of individual members; yet if they focus on the rights or needs of particular members, the result may be the weakening or disintegration of the family. Those who advocate regarding the family as the unit of care believe that what is best for the individuals and what is best for the family are generally the same or at least are not in conflict. But sometimes, as in this case, familial and individual interests do not appear to coincide. Thus, if Sharon is concerned primarily with preserving the mother's trust and the integrity of the family, she may be putting the children at significant risk. On the other hand, if her primary concern is the control of David's asthma, regularly scheduled meals and bedtimes for all the children, and an alternative to beatings as a way of dealing with Linda's stealing, her testimony in court may help weaken the integrity of the family.

This is an extremely difficult issue, and it is impossible to take a position that is beyond question or controversy. Nonetheless, we are inclined to agree with Goldstein, Freud, and Solnit that a policy of minimum coercive intervention by the state is most in accord with individual freedom, human dignity, and the intricate developmental processes of children: "So long as a child is a member of a functioning family, his paramount interest lies in the preservation of his family."[36] But where the dynamics of particular family interactions place the child at risk of serious bodily injury inflicted by the parents or the parents have repeatedly failed to prevent the child from suffering serious injury, there are grounds for intervention. One restriction on state intervention in such cases, however, is that the state must also be able to provide a better situation for the child. "If the state cannot or will not provide something better, even if it did not know this at the time the action was initiated, the least detrimental alternative would be to let the *status quo* persist, however unsatisfactory that might be."[37]

The question in Case 3.10 is how severe will the long-run negative consequences of the lack of regularity in their home life be to all the Trice children, and what are the special risks to David because of his asthma and to Linda because of her stealing and the subsequent beatings? If, on the basis of her knowledge of the situation, Sharon believes that one or more of these alternatives poses a significant risk of lasting harm to the children *and* if the state is able to provide something better, she should advise the court to intervene. If, on the other hand, *both* of these conditions are not met, she should not advise the court to intervene. Furthermore, if intervention is advisable, the less extreme alternative—placing the children in an institution that offers family therapy and the possibility of family reintegration—is, at least initially, preferable to options requiring more lasting separation.

Notes

1. By "parentalism" we mean what is conventionally referred to in the literature as "paternalism." But since women are no less capable than men of occupying the "paternal" or "father knows best" role in their dealings with others, we prefer the sexually neutral term.
2. This case has been provided by Peggy Jones, B.S.N., Community Health Nurse, Lansing, Michigan.
3. An important distinction can be drawn between "parentalism" *as a social practice* having certain roles and expectations governing the behavior of patients and health professionals in the total health care system and parentalism *as a justification for particular acts* of manipulation or coercion on the part of health professionals. Unless otherwise indicated, we use the term "parentalism" in the second sense.
4. James Childress, "Paternalism and Health Care," in Wade L. Robison and Michael S. Pritchard, eds., *Medical Responsibility* (Clifton, N.J.: Humana Press, 1979), p. 18.
5. As Charles Fried puts it, "even if the ends are the patient's own ends, to treat him as a means to them is to undermine his humanity insofar as humanity consists in choosing and being able to judge one's own ends, rather than being a machine which is used to serve ends, even one's own ends." Charles Fried, *Medical Experimentation: Personal Integrity and Social Policy* (Amsterdam: North Holland, 1974), p. 101.
6. *Ibid.*, p. 95.
7. This case has been provided by Bruce Walters, student in the College of Human Medicine at Michigan State University.
8. See Bruce Miller, "Autonomy and the Refusal of Lifesaving Treatment," *Hastings Center Report*, 11 (in press, 1981).
9. H. L. A. Hart, *Law, Liberty, and Morality* (New York: Vintage, 1966), p. 32–34.
10. John Stuart Mill, *On Liberty* (New York: Library of Liberal Arts, 1956), p. 117.
11. Childress, p. 24.
12. Gerald Dworkin, "Paternalism," *Monist*, 56 (January, 1972), p. 76f.
13. Kirsten Bennett in Case 3.2 might thus be criticized for not having worked harder at obtaining consent from Mr. Henry, during his lucid periods, to his being restrained, if necessary, in the future. The case, as presented, suggests that she may have been more concerned with securing his family's consent than his own.
14. Ultimately this condition must be modified to account for subjects who will never recover their capacity for rational reflection.
15. See Chapter 5, Section 1, Part B, for a further account of the role of the primary nurse.
16. This case has been provided by Bruce Walters.

17. Lawrence Stern, "Freedom, Blame, and the Moral Community," *Journal of Philosophy*, LXXI (February 14, 1974), p. 75.
18. *Ibid.*, p. 74.
19. Raymond Williams, *Keywords* (New York: Oxford, 1976), p. 156.
20. Stern, p. 76.
21. For an account of eight such ways, see Roderick M. Chisholm and Thomas D. Feehan, "The Intent to Deceive," *Journal of Philosophy, * LXXIV (March, 1977), pp. 143–159.
22. Irving M. Copi, *Introduction to Logic* (New York: Macmillan, 1978), p. 114.
23. Martin Benjamin, "Moral Agency and Negative Acts in Medicine," Wade L. Robison and Michael S. Pritchard, *Medical Responsibility* (Clifton, N.J.: Humana Press, 1979), pp. 169–180.
24. Anthony Shaw, "Dilemmas of 'Informed Consent' in Children," *New England Journal of Medicine, * 289 (October 25, 1973), p. 885.
25. *Ibid., * 886.
26. St. Augustine, *The Enchiridion*, quoted in Sissela Bok, *Lying: Moral Choice in Public and Private Life* (New York: Pantheon, 1978), p. 32.
27. Immanuel Kant, *Doctrine of Virtue*, quoted in Bok, p. 32.
28. Immanuel Kant, "On a Supposed Right to Lie from Altruistic Motives," excerpted in Bok, p. 269.
29. Alan Donagan, *The Theory of Morality* (Chicago: University of Chicago Press, 1977), p. 89.
30. Bok, p. 26f.
31. *Ibid.*, p. 223.
32. Lewis Thomas, *The Lives of a Cell* (New York: Viking, 1974), pp. 81–86.
33. Bok, p. 63.
34. Howard Brody, *Placebos and the Philosophy of Medicine* (Chicago: University of Chicago Press, 1980), pp. 25–44, 96–114.
35. This case is a variation of one reported in Kathleen A. Mahon and Sally J. Everson, "Moral Outrage—Nurse's Right or Responsibility: Ethics Rounds for Nurses," *Journal of Continuing Education*, 10 (No. 3, 1979), p. 4.
36. Joseph Goldstein, Anna Freud, and Albert J. Solnit, *Before the Best Interests of the Child* (New York: The Free Press, 1979), p. 5.
37. *Ibid.*, p. 21.

4

Recurring Ethical Issues
in Nurse-Physician Relationships

1. Conflicts between nurse and physician

Conflicts arise when either the nurse or the physician disagrees with the other's professional practice. In some situations the nurse believes that the physician's orders or actions result in poor care or are unsafe; in other instances the physician believes that the nurse's activities are similarly wrong. The following is an example of a conflict resulting from a nurse's assessment of a need for immediate medical care.

4.1 The doctor won't come

After working eight years as a nurse in an emergency room in a medium-sized city and in an inner-city hospital pediatric unit, Jackie Nardi presently is charge staff nurse two afternoons a week on a sixteen-bed pediatric unit in a community hospital.

Six-year-old Laurie Thoma was a new diabetic who, in Jackie's judgment, was close to a respiratory arrest. Jackie first phoned the resident on call, who happened to be new to the hospital. When he arrived, he was not only younger than Jackie but seemed to be uncertain of himself. Jackie gave him some suggestions regarding immediate medical care for Laurie, but according to her, "He just threw it down the tubes because I'm the nurse and he's the doctor." Then he left, saying he'd return after dinner.

Meanwhile, Jackie still believed it was a life-threatening situation to the

*child and called the pediatrician, Dr. Bauerlein, who was working in the
hospital emergency room. When he learned that the resident had been there
moments earlier, he refused to come. Jackie was frustrated: "I could see
Laurie's condition worsening. I could see a lot of things that needed to be
done, but I couldn't do anything about it because I can't write orders." She
thought Laurie needed more than her observations and decisions, so she
started calling Dr. Bauerlein every five minutes. She also called her supervisor
and convinced her that Dr. Bauerlein had to come immediately. Finally, the
supervisor went to the emergency room and brought him over. He was angry
at Jackie for her persistent calls; but he ordered, basically, the medical care
Jackie had suggested earlier to the resident.*

*Although Jackie never regretted getting emergency help for Laurie, she
dislikes the way Dr. Bauerlein now treats her. At times when a resident or
another nurse, especially her supervisor, is within hearing distance, he asks
Jackie medical questions relating to his various patients—questions he knows
she cannot, without a medical education and pediatric background like his,
answer correctly.*

This case raises a number of questions: What should a nurse's responsibility
be in making medical decisions (in the technical sense)? What should a nurse
do when her well-grounded recommendations are ignored? What, if anything,
should a nurse do when she disagrees with a physician's actions or lack of
action? The easiest solution for Jackie, of course, would have been simply to
wait for the doctor and follow his orders; but the result, if her assessment of
Laurie's precarious situation was correct, might have been Laurie's death.
Jackie's awareness of the medical situation placed her in an acute conflict
between complying with Dr. Bauerlein's wishes to be left alone and meeting
Laurie's need, as Jackie saw it, for emergency medical care.

Several factors contribute to tension in this and similar situations. Among
them are: the historical legacy of nurse-physician relationships, the expanding
scope of nursing practice, the socioeconomic and educational distance between nursing and medical professionals, and the ideology of professionalism
in nursing. Since these factors often impede or distort efforts to engage in
ethical inquiry, it is important to have some understanding of them.

A. Historical legacy

During the earliest period of nursing history, nursing and medicine developed
independently and had little contact until recognition of the medical value of
bedside nursing brought them together in the late eighteenth century. With

the development of the modern hospital came the introduction of the trained nurse, and patterns of relationships in hospitals developed that affect current nurse-physician relationships.[1] Physicians developed the medical staff; but as a part of that staff, they were not employed by, subordinate to, or responsible to the hospital administration. Physicians could and did, however, issue orders directly to nurses. The nursing staff position was quite different from that of the medical staff. Nurses were employed by, subordinate to, and directly responsible to the administration. Thus, nursing developed under the dual command of physicians and hospital administrators. Even today, the two lines of authority severely limit and complicate the decision-making role of a hospital nurse.[2]

The Nightingale plan for nursing schools, which included instruction in both scientific principles and practical experience, appeared in the United States in 1873. Unfortunately for American nursing, the schools had no endowment or financial backing, and hospitals quickly seized the opportunity to gain inexpensive student nurse labor. Nursing education was essentially an apprenticeship, and as late as the 1930s student nurses received little formal instruction in some hospitals.[3]

Under the dominance of male doctors and administrators, schools of nursing grew; and they were not noted for their development of independent, thoughtful nurses. Students entered nursing schools already expecting that women would defer to men, and therefore, that nurses would defer to doctors. Adding to the traditional subordination of nurses to physicians, nursing school faculties often culled out overly questioning and rebellious students.[4] The students' socialization and education taught them to be deferential. Many diploma schools included the study of textbooks such as L. J. Morison's *Steppingstones to Professional Growth,* published in a revised edition in 1965, which tells the student to cultivate loyalty, prudence, willingness, and cooperation since the physician has the right to expect such qualities. Further, the nurse must follow orders and uphold the physician's professional reputation.[5] Expected by society and trained by the nursing school to act as subordinates, most nurses behaved accordingly.

Yet tradition and nursing education alone cannot be blamed for the dominance of physicians and the deference of nurses. Beatrice and Philip Kalisch argue that a physician who sees himself as an independent, omnipotent man with mystical healing powers relates to co-workers as he does to patients and therefore insists that nurses and other health providers serve him in his "so-called captain of the ship role."[6]

The relegation of nursing to the subordinate position in the nurse-physician relationship has limited collaboration between the two professions. Empirical studies show that physicians are at the center of the decision-making process and that nurses carry out those decisions.[7] Further, psychiatrist Leonard Stein has described nurse-physician relationships in terms of a doctor-nurse game in which a nurse must appear to be passive. In this game any suggestion a nurse makes to a doctor must be masked in such a way as to seem as if it were his idea, and a doctor may not openly seek advice from a nurse.[8] The historical legacy of nurse-physician relationships, while affecting specific nurses and doctors in various ways, gives decision-making power to a doctor, requires passivity (or biting one's lip) of a nurse. If a nurse and a physican deviate from this pattern, the exchange of information and recommendations must occur in such a way that the doctor still appears to lead, the nurse to follow.

In Case 4.1, Jackie was the obvious loser in the doctor-nurse game with both doctors, the resident and Dr. Bauerlein. The new resident rejected Jackie's recommendations because, as she said, he was the doctor and she the nurse—a statement that indicates that she was well aware of the usual rules of the doctor-nurse game. Jackie forgot or ignored important rules by aggressively and publicly seeking out Dr. Bauerlein. The doctor, however, from the evidence of his later attempts to belittle or embarrass her, clearly remembered the game and placed importance on the rule that he must, as the doctor, be treated as the leader who needed no obvious assistance from her. If they continue their relationship in this historically spawned, stereotypical manner, the game effectively limits their communication, and Jackie has little chance of involving Dr. Bauerlein in an investigation of their overlapping roles and responsibilities as colleagues. In addition, had the resident and Jackie not been involved in the doctor-nurse game, the situation probably would never have developed into a problem. If Jackie and the resident had been able to exchange information freely and examine each other's ideas about Laurie's treatment, the resident would have been quick to recognize the validity of Jackie's suggestions.

B. The expanding scope of nursing practice

In some clinical situations, as in Case 4.1, a nurse believes she can correctly diagnose and treat a particular problem in an emergency, but she is not allowed legally to act upon her knowledge. In another kind of situation, it is not the nurse but the physician who wants the nurse to perform activities that are legally prohibited, such as making rounds and prescribing postoperative medications. Thus, to carry out tasks that are outside the scope of professional nursing practice sometimes requires the nurse to break the law.

However, the line between medicine and nursing is blurred and in some complex medical procedures and institutional organizations, it is difficult for a doctor and nurse to differentiate tasks that are strictly medical from those that are legitimately within the realm of nursing.[9]

The expansion of knowledge, together with the technological and social changes that have occurred rapidly in the last quarter-century, have necessitated redefinitions of the scope of nursing practice and have contributed to tensions in nurse-physician relationships. Such changes include the use of life-maintenance machines, automatic clinical laboratory equipment, computers, complex medical interventions, artificial replacements of human parts, human transplants, and resulting specialization within both medicine and nursing.[10] Among the many social changes affecting the scope of nursing practice are increased social mobility; increased pluralism of religion, culture, race, and age among patient populations seeking care; and increased concern for good health among certain groups as evidenced by interest in physical fitness, health foods, alternative care plans for childbirth, alternative health care providers in addition to physicians, and new health care systems such as health maintenance organizations. Given these technological and social changes, certain nurses, through in-service education, college or university courses, independent study, or experience, may know more about some aspect of a particular treatment or apparatus or machine than do the physicians with whom they work. For example, an experienced and knowledgeable nurse working full time in an intensive care unit may know more about certain treatments in that unit than a physician working there only briefly during his educational program. In addition, nurses, who usually spend more time with patients than physicians, often know considerably more about their patients' strengths, weaknesses, desires, and needs than do some physicians, who may see patients only during short visits. Furthermore, some nurses, in viewing nursing as a "caring" more than a "curing" profession, see health education needs as important and as requiring more professional time and effort than that allotted in some medical treatment programs that focus on specific disease processes. In response to pressures to clarify the expanding role of nursing, in recent years nearly all states have attempted to redefine the scope of nursing practice.

In 1955 the American Nurses' Association approved a model definition of nursing practice that prohibited nurses from performing any medical act. Yet nursing education had already been strengthened to the extent that nurses were making diagnostic and therapeutic decisions in providing nursing care; the disclaimers that they were not to do so were out of date at the time that various states incorporated the model definition into their practice acts.

During the fifties and sixties, nursing functions continued to expand into the overlapping areas of medical and nursing practice. Pressure from both within and without the nursing profession mounted, and legal changes came rapidly in the seventies. Between 1971 and 1975, thirty states amended their nursing practice acts to legitimize diagnosis and treatment by nurses, and the trend has continued. The movement to develop new legal definitions of nursing practice is related directly to the need to legalize advanced nursing practice.[11]

Nurses, depending upon their state of residence, may or may not practice under a nursing practice act that allows them to carry out nursing diagnosis and treatment and/or medical diagnosis and treatment. They may live in a state that requires special certification or agency protocols, rules, and procedures before they engage in diagnosis and treatment. In some states, diagnosis and treatment functions must be delegated to nurses. In others, nurses may be absolutely prohibited from diagnosing and prescribing treatments. Finally, in some states, regulations and broad definitions only vaguely differentiate nursing diagnosis and treatment from medical diagnosis and treatment.

Given this variety, and changes in legal definitions of the scope of nursing practice, it is understandable that physicians and nurses may disagree or be confused as to the legality of nurses' performing diagnostic and treatment procedures. As discussed in Chapter 1, before engaging in ethical inquiry the nurse needs to have the facts about a given situation clearly in mind, and the scope of nursing practice as defined in the state practice act is one such fact. Unless nurses keep themselves informed and educate other health workers in their community concerning current revisions of their state practice acts, nurses and physicians are likely to view the nurses' functions from conflicting and perhaps erroneous points of view. Nevertheless, ethical inquiry into conflicts between nurse and physician may be impeded by disagreements about the nurse's rightful functions even though both the nurse and the physician may be aware of their state practice acts and related rules and regulations. This is especially true if the acts or rules are open to broad interpretation or if the physician and nurse disagree about the scope of nursing thus described.

To return again to Case 4.1, both Jackie's recognition of legal constraints on her practice as a nurse and her perception of the scope of nursing practice, which differed from that of Dr. Bauerlein, influenced their relationship. Although Jackie is currently a registered nurse with eight years' experience, she did not have the required additional education for certification as an advanced nurse practitioner. Legally, according to her state's nursing practice act, she could not medically treat Laurie. When both persons authorized by law to provide medical help for Laurie chose not to act, Jackie enlisted the help of her nurse supervisor, but she also kept calling persistently herself. Jackie clearly demonstrated that since she recognized she could not treat Laurie herself, she had to get help from a doctor. Thus, the conflict between Jackie and Dr. Bauerlein was affected not only by the historical legacy of the health professions in the form of the doctor-nurse game and her failure in that game, but also by the scope of her duties as determined by her state's current nursing practice act.

We are not suggesting that the public should have no legal protection from unqualified health providers. Nurses, such as Jackie, must recognize the general value of practice acts and observe their constraints. Nonetheless, at times the nurse must override a practice act, as she might any law in the name of a more stringent moral obligation. Note that no matter what the practice act stated about a nurse's making a diagnosis, Jackie disregarded that issue when she observed Laurie and decided that the child was in a life-threatening situation. Dr. Bauerlein's later attempts to discredit Jackie's ability to think for herself indicate that he thinks nurses should not diagnose. Quite simply, Dr. Bauerlein and Jackie did not agree as to the scope of Jackie's nursing practice.

Jackie, believing that her responsibility to get immediate help for Laurie fell within the scope of her nursing practice, did not obey Dr. Bauerlein and stop calling him; rather, she persisted until he came to the unit. Certainly, the nursing practice act did not forbid her from aggressively seeking his services. The tradition that the nurse should obey the doctor automatically is in conflict with the conception of a nurse who thinks for herself when she has strong grounds for evaluating a particular diagnosis and course of treatment. Yet time-worn attitudes linger in both professions. They are seen in a physician who expects a nurse's unconditional obedience and in parallel form in a nurse who hesitates to disagree with a physician even when she has good reason to do so. The following case presents a nurse in conflict between obeying or acting upon her own diagnosis and treatment plans.

4.2 Orders not to teach

Fran Hilkenmeyer, fifty-one-year-old clinical supervisor for South Lake Community College student nurses, has observed a mastectomy patient who, in her assessment, needs instruction. However, as was true of several other mastectomy patients she has seen recently at Mercy Hospital, the team of physicians that did the surgery does not want the nurses to teach the patient exercises for the affected arm. When Fran asked the head nurse why, she did not receive a clear answer and learned only that the doctors do not want special rehabilitation groups to come to the hospital to talk to their patients. Fran knows that nurses in many hospitals offer classes to promote the recovery of post-mastectomy patients.

Fran says she "feels strongly about the woman." She sees that the patient needs help, but she has not questioned the physicians about their orders that there be no teaching because "I don't know the physicians well enough to meet them head-on. I'm sure my hesitation goes back to my earlier ideas about not questioning doctors, which I don't really believe in any more but which just crop up every once in a while. I happen to think very highly of the surgeons involved. If I were to have surgery, they would be the ones I would go to. I hate to question them because I know they are good. When I get the chance, I do a bit of relationship building with them, and I will probably face them with the question before very long. My courage is mounting."

Fran, a graduate almost three decades ago of a major university school of nursing, was inclined to act in conflicting ways by the historical legacy of the nursing profession, which inculcated a deferential role, and by her recognition of the expanded scope of contemporary professional nursing. She saw the importance of being assertive and acting upon her diagnosis; yet, she held back. She chose not to attempt to instruct mastectomy patients until she herself talked with the surgeons, which would probably not occur until after this particular woman had left the hospital. She hopes, of course, to obtain their approval of her plans for teaching; however, her hopes are probably unrealistic since these physicians have allowed no other nurses to instruct their patients. In attempting to define the problem, Fran asked only one question: "Should I approach the physicians with my questions?" An underlying question, which she did not explicitly identify, was, "If the physicians say that they do not want me or any other nurse or student nurse to teach their patients, should I proceed to teach without their approval or against their wishes?" By focusing attention on the first question, Fran may ignore ethical inquiry into the underlying question of whether nurses should be obedient to physicians.

Before continuing the discussion of obedience, two remaining major factors need to be examined since a combination of factors simultaneously contributes to tension in many nurse-physician conflicts.

C. Socioeconomic and educational distance between nursing and medical professionals

Until recently, access to medical education was generally limited to white males of upper-middle-class family backgrounds,[12] which meant that physicians, as a group, had higher social-class backgrounds than nurses, as a group. In addition, the unequal incomes of the two professions have allowed physicians to remain in a much higher socioeconomic class than most nurses. With disparity of income come differences in values and styles of life; thus nurses and physicians tend to live in different neighborhoods and socialize in different groups. Of course, people do not have to be best friends to work congenially and effectively together, but they must be able to share important information with one another. Empirical studies, however, show that nurses and physicians are not sharing colleagues; rather, they work side by side with severely limited communication and minimal interaction.[13]

In Case 4.2, Fran's problem in overcoming the communication gap between herself and the physicians, whom she viewed as highly competent, is no different from problems experienced by other nurses, some much younger, less experienced, and less well-educated than Fran. Nurses, generally, have less formal education than physicians. Nursing education for registered nurses requires two, three, or four years of study in a nursing school; for some nurses, nursing education includes an additional one to two years in a master's level graduate program, and for a still smaller number of nurses the educational program includes several more years in a doctoral program. Medical education for doctors of medicine and osteopathy usually includes three to four years of college study, three to four years of medical school, a one-year internship, and, for most physicians, two to four years in a residency program. In simple numbers, educational programs for most nurses last two to four years while educational programs for most doctors extend from nine to thirteen years, although professionals in both groups engage in lifelong education. Needless to say, medicine remains a more prestigious and powerful profession than nursing.

D. The ideology of professionalism in nursing

In recent years nurses have intensified their efforts to gain a higher level of professionalism; but the process has been and continues to be stressful. Although some nurses have felt threatened, other nurses have gained support and courage from positions nursing leaders have taken concerning various professional nursing issues, such as the goal that baccalaureate nursing education be the minimum preparation for the professional nurse as outlined by the American Nurses' Association in 1965. The ANA position linked professionalism to baccalaureate preparation at a time when over 88 percent of the 582,000 employed registered nurses were diploma graduates.[14] Since that time, the shift of nursing education from diploma programs operated by hospitals to two-year associate degree programs in community colleges and four-year baccalaureate degree programs in colleges and universities has continued. Yet, ten years later, 81 percent of an estimated 906,000 employed registered nurses had less than a baccalaureate nursing education, and pressure within the nursing profession for individual nurses to return to college for baccalaureate and master's degrees in nursing remains strong.[15]

Reflecting this drive for more education, recognition, and higher professional status, many in nursing have tried to enrich nursing's conception of itself. But, according to Marlene Kramer's research, students who enter nursing schools continue to hold outdated conceptions about nursing; and they leave school still believing that "real" nursing is *only* bedside nursing.[16] Nevertheless, many nurses think that nursing must develop a more complex self-conception and move beyond the "downstairs maid" image symbolized by the nurse's uniform, which Dorothy Mereness once described as a house dress complete with dustcap. To Carol Garant,

"Real" nurses do not necessarily wear white uniforms and caps, carry lamps or long stemmed roses at graduation, give bedpans, bed baths, injections, and enemas or "push" pills. "Real" nurses also engage in research, deliver babies, teach health, do group and individual psychotherapy, work with drug addicts, administer anesthesia, own their own mental health centers, and "hang out shingles" in private practice. "Real" nurses also diagnose patients and clients—no longer do they *presume* patients to be dead or are their clients *thought* to be pregnant. "Real" nurses use their brains as well as their hands and feet.[17]

Garant's "real" nurse relates directly to the nurse practitioner model of practice, which is now firmly established. In 1978 fifty-three collegiate schools offered 103 master's level special and general nurse practitioner programs.[18] The expanded role of nursing, in providing nurse practitioners with both a wider range of activities and an acknowledged role in decision-making, offers meaningful incentives to other nurses to acquire new skills and a means for upward mobility in clinical nursing practice. Thus, while the nurse practitioner model of practice may only change the economic distance between medicine and nursing slightly, it reduces some of the social and educational distance between the two professions, both through the nurse's clinical experiences and formal education and through her exhibition of clinical skills that demand recognition. But while particular physicians may respect an individual nurse's expertise and judgment, the struggle for the control of nursing continues. It can be seen at the national level, for example, in the split between the ANA and the American Academy of Pediatrics over pediatric nurse practitioner certification.[19]

Also supporting a more up-to-date conception of nursing, as described above, are social changes related to the women's movement. While most nurses continue to isolate themselves from the women's movement, and while some feminists have, at times, rejected nursing because of its stereotypical handmaiden image, nursing has profited from the movement.[20] In clarifying the use of sexist language, feminists have helped underscore the increasing awareness of nurses that the professional image of a thoughtful, independent, well-educated, responsible nurse is incompatible with the image implied by references to staff nurses as "the girls" or "the kids" or by physicians' requests prefaced by "Hey, honey."

Conflicts between nurses and physicians arise, at times, when a nurse tries to gain and use increased skills and education or responds to interactions from a feminist point of view. To return to "Orders Not to Teach," Fran acknowledged her acceptance of the ideology of professionalism in nursing when she said she no longer believed that the doctors must not be questioned and by her obvious concern that the patient needed instruction which, she believed, she was prepared to give. Yet this did not automatically lead her out of the deferent role or convince her at once that teaching the patient was legitimately within the scope of her nursing practice; nor did it instantly convince her that she must bridge the communication gap between herself and the physicians.

In summary, nurse-physician conflicts are affected by the historical legacy of the health professions, the expanding scope of nursing practice, the socio-economic and educational distance between nurses and doctors, and the ideology of professionalism in nursing. Although these are not all the factors involved in such relationships (and they overlap in many respects), they are major sources of tensions. These tensions at times not only contribute to nurse-physician conflicts but block ethical inquiry into them.

2. Obedience

The question, "Should a nurse always obey a physician?" arose in both cases previously described in this chapter and is a central concern in the following case.

4.3 Disagreement with a feeding order

Cheryl Pulec worked during her last two years in school as a nursing assistant on a gynecology floor in a large university medical center and has had six months experience in a neonatal intensive care unit as a registered nurse. When the unit is busy, she cares for two babies; but she has cared for only one baby, Matthew Brenner, since his admission a week ago.

Last night, one of the residents wrote orders to start feeding Matthew and then left the unit. When Cheryl read them, she thought they were "crazy orders" since they included "giving sterile water over twenty-four hours." She had never seen such a beginning feeding order, and she was concerned about possible fluid and electrolyte problems. She told another resident in the unit her grounds for objecting and that she felt uneasy about beginning Matthew's feeding according to that plan. Nevertheless, he told her to proceed according to the written orders.

Even though directed by two doctors to start the feedings, Cheryl thought that since she still disagreed with the feeding plan, she would not begin it. She liked her staff nurse position and tried to do a good job, which included, of course, carrying out medical orders and working well with the doctors; but she thought Matthew's well-being was more important than the possible repercussions she might suffer for her efforts to get the orders changed and her refusal to carry them out. Therefore, she considered whether she should approach a third resident and repeat her reasons for not wanting to carry out the feeding order.

Ms. Pulec's reasons for acting in this situation are based on her obligations to Matthew as a health care provider, to the hospital as an employee, and to the physicians as a co-worker. When she became a registered nurse, she assumed an obligation to provide safe, effective, and morally responsible care to her clients. Therefore, she has a duty to do her best for Matthew Brenner. She is well within her legal obligations, as defined by the state nursing practice act and her contract with the hospital, to question any medical order and to refrain from implementing it if, in her judgment, the order is unsafe. Nevertheless, since nurses have traditionally obeyed physicians, she recognizes that the physicians expect her to carry out the orders as a part of the traditional nursing role. Finally, Ms. Pulec believes she must act so as to maintain her self-respect as an autonomous, thoughtful, reliable person.

Ms. Pulec has time to make a thoughtful decision since the risk to Matthew is very slight if she delays the feedings briefly. The question is: Will

Matthew be harmed by the feedings in any significant or lasting way? Given Ms. Pulec's limited experience—she has been employed in the neonatal intensive care unit for only six months—her opposition to the feedings perhaps should not be given the weight of the two resident physicians' decision in favor of the sterile water feedings since they have had more education and clinical experience than she. Her apparent lack of experience, however, is offset by her scientific education regarding fluids and electrolytes, her study of other babies during her employment, and her acute awareness of Matthew's needs since he has been the only baby in her care during the past week. It is possible that the first physician wrote the order while thinking not specifically of Matthew but of babies generally, and that the second physician, not seeing a gross error in the feeding order, elected to let the orders stand. Given the second physician's decision not to act, and given that Ms. Pulec based her decision on her brief nursing experience and on the negative evidence that the order was wrong because she had never seen any like it, she could conclude that the feeding order might be within the limits of acceptable medical practice, even if it were not ideal. Therefore, she might proceed without causing Matthew undue harm. But even though the feedings are probably not unsafe, Ms. Pulec is convinced that they are not best for Matthew since they may upset his fluid and electrolyte balance.

Ms. Pulec's obligations to Matthew and the physicians are in conflict. She cannot obey the orders and thus act as a loyal subordinate to the physicians in the traditional sense and simultaneously meet Matthew's needs as she has defined them. But a nurse's primary obligations, in the end, are to clients, not physicians. The reason a nurse works with a physician and his medical treatment plan is to help provide a client with the best possible health care.[21] Whatever the strength of the historical legacy and the dominating status of medicine, whenever a nurse faces a choice between obligation to a physician and obligation to a client, she must recognize that her obligation to a client is primary. In Ms. Pulec's case, her obligation to the physicians is clearly secondary to, and based upon, her obligation to the baby; and the choice of overriding the obligation to the physicians carries only a small risk. While Ms. Pulec may lose her reputation as a congenial worker, Matthew has much to gain if, in fact, a different feeding order would be better for him.

Ms. Pulec's situation, like other situations in which a nurse considers alternatives to what a physician has ordered, rests at some point on a wide "spectrum of urgency," that is, on a continuum of cases in which the available time to make decisions varies. The spectrum begins at one end with problems that may be solved at a leisurely pace, allowing time for reflection, collection of further data, debate, and discussion, and ends at the other end with urgent questions that demand quick solutions and immediate actions. The low-urgency end of the spectrum includes such situations as those in which a physician and nurse disagree about the correct answer to a question that a young pregnant woman asks in trying to decide if she should choose a home delivery attended by a midwife or a hospital delivery attended by a physician. In such a situation, the physician, nurse, and client have several months to study and to debate all aspects of the situation. The high-urgency end of the spectrum includes emergency situations in which a physician and a nurse disagree about an order for actions that must be carried out immediately. For example, a nurse and a physician may choose to allocate care differently for three accident victims admitted simultaneously to an emergency room.

The "spectrum of urgency" can be used as a guideline for nurses who question a physician's orders in situations involving practices that fall within the range of generally acceptable medical care. In situations in which urgency is low, when ample time is available for reasonable reflection and discussion, a rule-utilitarian argument (See Chapter 2, Section 2, Part A) that nurses obey doctors as the best course of action to insure the best overall outcome for clients is much less strong than in emergency situations. To return to Case 4.3, if Ms. Pulec agrees with the utilitarian goal of the greatest happiness for the largest number of patients, a goal supported by many hospitals in numerous policies, she might agree that she should be obedient and follow all physicians' orders that appear to fall within the broad range of acceptable practice, including the feeding order that a second physician supported. She could conclude that all nurses should follow all such physicians' orders because most of the time the orders would be correct; the greatest number of persons would thus be effectively served.

Two problems with this argument, however, immediately come to light. First, physicians' orders, like all human judgments, are sometimes wrong. If a nurse blindly followed all of them, harm to the patient could result, as the research study in Chapter 1 illustrated. Thus, insofar as a nurse has an obligation to follow a doctor's orders, it is only a prima facie obligation and may be overridden in certain circumstances by other factors. A nurse must be careful not to confuse a well-grounded prima facie obligation with blind faith. Second, nurses who operate under such a regime may become automatons, unable to make the responsible decisions that are necessary for high-quality nursing care. Thus, while in the short run the result might seem to be the greatest happiness for the greatest number of patients, over the long run, the harm to some patients and the poor quality of care delivered by automatons would significantly compromise overall happiness. The idea that nurses should obey physicians, when examined in low-urgency cases, appears to have little to be said for it apart from appeals to tradition.

The nearer a case is to the other end of the spectrum, the greater the need for a nurse to follow a physician's orders without debate. In general, a physician's medical expertise should be greater than a nurse's medical expertise since a nursing education, by its very nature, focuses upon nursing rather than medicine. In most emergency situations the greatest number of satisfactory outcomes for clients will occur if a nurse refrains from blocking acceptable orders and cooperates in delivering quick efficient help, although she might judge that a particular course is not the one that she believes would be best. The main goal in a crisis is to provide adequate help quickly, and this goal would obviously be blocked by lengthy debate and discussion. In a cool moment after the crisis has passed, the nurse should engage the physician in a discussion regarding the feasibility and worth of alternative actions which may have been more appropriate. A nurse, especially an experienced nurse, may be more knowledgeable than a physician about a specific client, situation, or procedure. Through calm, rational discussion the nurse and the physician might learn from each other and agree how best to manage similar crises in the future.

Although a nurse generally presumes that a physician is right in an emergency situation, there are nonetheless limits to what can reasonably be presumed. When the medical care a physician orders clearly constitutes unacceptable practice, a nurse is obligated to disobey orders. For example, an emergency room nurse and a resident physician disagreed about whether the use of a local anesthetic was acceptable practice in the case of a five-year-old girl who had suffered a huge vaginal laceration. After the doctor had ordered the nurse to pry the terrified and wildly struggling girl's legs apart while he repeatedly tried but failed to inject a local anesthetic, the nurse, believing that such treatment was unacceptable because of the child's fear and pain and the size of the laceration, refused to continue assisting the physician. She demanded that another resident physician be called, which resulted in the child being taken to surgery and given a general anesthetic.[22] Given the psychic trauma caused the girl by repeated attempts to repair the laceration, further efforts in the emergency room clearly fell outside of the bounds of acceptable practice.

In summary, if an order for action is clearly outside acceptable medical practice, a nurse should not obey it even in an emergency and should seek safe care for the client from another source as did the emergency room nurse in the previous example. If a physician's order is within the wide range of acceptable practice and time is pressing, the nurse should obey that order, even if she would prefer another course of action, and she should discuss the matter with the physician later.[23] At the lower levels of the spectrum of urgency—and most medical care allows some time for consideration—the nurse should calmly and rationally discuss with the physician those orders that she questions, including orders that fall within the wide range of acceptable medical practice, in order to provide the best possible care for each client. Given these guidelines, the nurse in the feeding order case, Ms. Pulec, should choose to approach a third resident, since he is readily available, and to repeat her reasons for not following the feeding order in the hope that he will cancel the order and write a new one.[24]

3. Conscientious refusal

Placing a situation somewhere along the spectrum of urgency suggests one way for a nurse to begin to reflect upon when to question a physician's order. Further, as the previous discussion indicates, a nurse has the duty to override a medical order that is clearly outside acceptable medical practice and that may jeopardize a client in some way. In the following case, the nurse based her decision on her medical knowledge, discounted the risk that her actions might jeopardize her position as a nurse, and followed her own judgment without hesitation.

4.4 Emergency room

When Valerie Workman graduated in 1965 from a university school of nursing, which she described as "an older school," she believed as she had been taught—when a doctor gives an order, follow it. But she no longer follows orders unquestioningly; she now questions doctors much more thoroughly, even though she recognizes that they often "aren't exactly thrilled that I question their judgment." In describing herself and other nurses, she says that, "the older we get, the wiser we get—sometimes."

In 1975, when Valerie was working in a hospital emergency room, Mrs. Brown, a twenty-four-year-old woman who was six months pregnant and in shock, was admitted following a serious automobile accident. The physician on duty was an older man whom Valerie did not feel was always competent in emergencies. Valerie, certain that the patient's life was in danger, suggested starting an IV, but the doctor rejected her suggestion. Alarmed, Valerie decided she must act, started the IV, initiated other emergency measures, and called for additional medical help. The physician was furious at Valerie's independent action, and she was extremely angry with him. Later, she remembers, she "got complete backing from other doctors" and the matter was dropped.

How did Valerie know not to accept the doctor's orders? Perhaps she reasoned that if a nurse believes that she has a moral obligation to meet a client's needs, then she must take risks, both by refusing to defer to a physician whose actions impede the delivery of adequate help and by taking independent emergency action. To Valerie, the young woman's chance to live must have seemed worth the risk to her own career. Had she chosen to obey orders, and had Mrs. Brown died, Valerie might not have been able to live with her conscience later.

The doctor's decision against the IV differed so radically from usual emergency treatment that the other physicians in the hospital agreed that Valerie and not the doctor had acted more appropriately. Moreover, since Valerie's action was justified on well-grounded medical and ethical considerations, she had no reason to defend her conduct simply by an appeal to conscience. A nurse may sometimes be in a situation, however, where what a physician does falls within acceptable medical practice and the nurse can justify a refusal to carry out an order or to participate in a procedure only on the basis of conscience. The following case focuses on what may be called "conscientious refusal."[25]

4.5 Amniocentesis to determine sex

Sylvia Hutton, a nurse practitioner with graduate-level education in genetics and counseling, is employed at the University Clinical Center. Among her many duties, she explains to women seeking amniocentesis (a procedure to obtain cells for fetal chromosome studies) what to expect during the procedure. After the results are known, she is the main person who meets with the woman and her husband to discuss the meaning of the findings. At times she meets with them alone; at other times she invites health team members with knowledge about the particular genetic problem facing the family to attend.

Generally, chromosome studies are done when parents, because of the mother's advanced age or a family history of a specific genetic condition, suspect that the fetus may be affected by the condition. Before joining the Clinical Center, Sylvia thought about the implications of such work, including the possibility that most women would choose abortion if tests indicated that a child might be mentally retarded. Until recently Sylvia opposed abortion, but she now believes that abortion is permissible for parents who recognize that they do not have the strength, support, or money to rear a handicapped child; and she believes that abortion in such cases may also be in the best interests of society, which must bear the cost of a person who will require a lifetime of care.

Susan Baker has asked for amniocentesis to determine the sex of her fetus. Susan and her husband have two healthy, normal sons and have decided that, given the cost of rearing children, they can afford only one more child. Specifically, they want a girl to balance their family, and they plan an immediate abortion if the fetus is male.

Dr. Milton Ely, who usually performs the amniocentesis procedures, believes that the Bakers are as entitled to choose abortion as any other family and that they have the same right as other families to ask for the technical information that can be obtained through amniocentesis. But Sylvia believes that the procedure is not justified: the family has the means to raise the third child, boy or girl, and the potential cost or gain to society is basically the same whatever the sex of the fetus. Sylvia believes that to do the amniocentesis and a possible abortion is frivolous; therefore, she has decided that she must refuse to participate in any way in determining the sex of the Baker fetus.

Sylvia's supervisor knows Sylvia's objections but has asked her to meet with the Bakers, offer support, and perform her duties as usual. Dr. Ely has told Sylvia that her refusal to participate will not influence the Bakers' decision in any way, so she may as well stop making a fuss. Sylvia is afraid that if she submits to pressure from her supervisor and Dr. Ely, she will have the death of a male fetus on her conscience and she will have to admit that she is just one more spineless, manipulable nurse who has no meaningful convictions.[26]

In order to explore the question of when a nurse should (or may) use an appeal to conscience to refuse to participate in a particular procedure, we need first to analyze the notion of an appeal to "conscience." For if appeals to conscience are to carry special weight, it is important to be able to distinguish them from appeals to self-interest, convenience, etc. In a discussion of appeals to conscience, James Childress cites three cases which illustrate that "Conscience is a mode of consciousness and thought about one's own acts and their value or disvalue."

1. On June 21, 1956, Arthur Miller, the playwright, appeared before the House Committee on Un-American Activities (HUAC) which was examining the unauthorized use of passports, and he was asked who had been present at meetings with Communist writers in New York City. "Mr. Chairman, I understand the

philosophy behind this question and I want you to understand mine. When I say this, I want you to understand that I am not protecting the Communists or the Communist Party. I am trying to, and I will, *protect my sense of myself.* I could not use the name of another person and bring trouble on him. . . . I ask you not to ask me that question. . . . All I can say, sir, is that *my conscience* will not permit me to use the name of another person."

2. On December 29, 1970, Governor Winthrop Rockefeller of Arkansas commuted to life imprisonment the death sentences of the fifteen prisoners then on death row. He said, "I cannot and will not turn my back on life-long Christian teachings and beliefs, merely to let history run out its course on a fallible and failing theory of punitive justice." Understanding his decision as "purely personal and philosophical," he insisted that the records of the prisoners were irrelevant to it. He continued, "I am aware that there will be reaction to my decision. However, failing to take this action while it is within my power, *I could not live with myself.*"

3. In late December, 1972, Captain Michael Heck refused to carry out orders to fly more bombing missions in Vietnam. He wrote his parents: "I've taken a very drastic step. I've refused to take part in this war any longer. *I cannot in good conscience* be a part of it." He also said, "I can live with prison easier than I can with taking part in the war." "I would refuse even a ground job supervising the loading of bombs or refueling aircraft. I cannot be a participant . . . *a man has to answer to himself first.*"[27]

In analyzing these cases, Childress suggests that an appeal to conscience is based on a desire to preserve one's integrity or wholeness as a person (see Chapter 1, Section 4, "Developing a Systematic Framework"). These conscientious refusers are predicting that if they were to act in certain ways they would betray themselves as being certain kinds of people having certain personal ideals and standards of conduct. Insofar as their conceptions of themselves as particular people are determined by having and abiding by certain standards of conduct, what is at stake is nothing less than personal identity.[28]

In addition, Childress suggests that appeals to conscience are personal and subjective, based on standards that one does not necessarily apply to others; founded on a prior judgment of rightness or wrongness, since conscience itself is not a criterion of rightness or wrongness; and motivated by personal sanction rather than external authority.[29] Sylvia's behavior in Case 4.5 seems to meet all of the conditions for making her act one of conscientious refusal. First, Sylvia spoke only for herself in this case. She did not attempt to imagine what another nurse or physician might think or feel about using amniocentesis to determine sex. Nor would she oppose or try to prevent some other nurse from performing her duties. Second, she judged that her participation would be wrong because amniocentesis for what she regarded as a trivial reason could lead to the abortion of a healthy fetus. Sylvia used her conscience as a guide only to the extent that she debated with herself; that is, when she debated with her conscience about whether she should participate or not. Sylvia's belief that the abortion of a healthy fetus for "trivial" reasons is morally wrong was the basis for her appeal to conscience. A "conflict-of-conscience" arose because, although she believed in general that parents have the right to choose abortion, she rejected the grounds for the decision in this particular case. The conflict here is similar to one that might be experienced by someone who endorses a strong interpretation of the right to freedom of speech while also being opposed to its being exercised to further the cause of Nazism. Third, Sylvia, like Miller, Rockefeller, and Heck in the three passages Childress cites, felt first and foremost answerable to herself (Miller: "I am trying to, and I will, protect my sense of myself"; Rockefeller: "I could not live with myself"; and Heck: "A man has to answer to himself first"). Sylvia believed that if she participated in the amniocentesis in any way she would have to acknowledge that she was a spineless person without the courage of her deepest convictions. Not only would she have felt guilt for the possible death of a healthy fetus, but she also would have felt ashamed of herself for not having had the strength to act in accord with her personal ideals of conduct—ideals that in part determine her identity.[30] The fact that her participation in this procedure is perfectly legal and that the act is not punishable by any external authority has no bearing whatever on her deliberations.

We may now turn to the general question of under what circumstances and for what reasons a nurse may appeal to her conscience and refuse to participate in a particular procedure. As the discussion of Case 4.5 indicated, a nurse may make an appeal to conscience as a last resort when she has exhausted all other arguments for justifying her action. The appeal to conscience is personal or subjective, although the moral standards on which it is based may or may not apply to other persons; it must *follow* a judgment of rightness or wrongness; and it must be based upon personal sanction rather than upon external authority. The individual nurse must determine the extent to which the act in question constitutes a rupture of her integrity or wholeness as a person or a particular self. Then she must determine whether the shame or "bad conscience" that would follow from her per-formance of the act constitutes a greater threat to her well-being than the possible punishment that may be forthcoming from whatever authority (agency or physician) may be displeased by her refusal. (A discussion of a nursing supervisor's response to a subordinate's appeal to conscience is included in Chapter 5.)

The question that the next case presents is whether a nurse's use of conscientious refusal is appropriate in a situation in which a physician's orders and a patient's wishes are in conflict.

4.6 Disagreeing with a full code order

Ms. Doris Winn, a staff nurse with two years experience in a cardiac care unit, strongly disagreed with Dr. Cunningham's full code order for Mr. Chester Saukin, an eighty-seven-year-old retired farmer with a history of three MIs and three years of cardiac failure. Ms. Winn believed Mr. Saukin was ready to die, for he had told her that was all he wanted. When she told Dr. Cunningham this, he simply walked away from her. She knew he always ordered full codes on all his patients. Ms. Winn understood, also, that legally she had to do the full code, but she thought it would be very hard for her.

Could Ms. Winn make an appeal to conscience and not carry out the full code order? Before discussing this question, we need to return to two earlier discussions, one concerning the spectrum of urgency and the other concerning medical decisions. When Mr. Saukin was first admitted, Ms. Winn acted as if the implied disagreement between Mr. Saukin's wishes and Dr. Cunningham's order for a full code fell on the lower end of the urgency spectrum. She had time to tell Dr. Cunningham of Mr. Saukin's statement that he was ready to die, even though the physician did not initially allow her to discuss her disagreement with the full code order. Dr. Cunningham's behavior indicated his belief that as a physician his order for the full code was indisputable. The question remains, is the decision for a full code a technical medical decision? If the answer is yes, then the nurse has little recourse; the physician's superior medical training gives him presumptive authority in technical medical decisions. But if the answer is no, that the decision for a full code is a decision in the medical context but not mainly a medical decision in the technical sense, the nurse may have something to contribute—especially when she has some reason to believe that the decision does not reflect the values and life plan of a conscious, competent adult.[31]

It is possible, however, that Dr. Cunningham's initial refusal to talk with Ms. Winn has resulted from his adherence to the letter of state law rather than from his denial of her possible contribution. The state where he and Ms. Winn practice has no "living will" legislation that would grant legal standing to a person's previously stated and documented opposition to certain kinds of intervention such as full codes when he or she is terminally ill.[32] Further, strictly speaking, there is no legal justification for a "no code," even though the practice is not uncommon and in some medical-legal communities is accepted as standard practice. However, according to a strict interpretation of current state law, "no codes" may be considered abandonment and possibly even murder.

Many people believe that the law in this context has not kept pace with advances in life-prolonging technology. Although a conscious, competent adult has the right to accept or refuse medical treatment, in most states this right disappears as soon as the person is no longer conscious and competent. Efforts to draft legislation in this area aim to insure that thoughtful directives with regard to life-prolonging medical intervention, made when one is conscious and competent, will be honored when one is no longer conscious and competent.

Ms. Winn strongly believes that such changes in the law are badly needed if the rights of patients are to remain in force toward the end of their lives. As she explained:

"I think patients should have the right to say if they want to live and if they want to die; I think that we, as nurses and doctors, should be able to respect that. We're all here to heal people, get them well, and send them home. And if we aren't able to do that, and the patient has suffered for a long time and wants to die, I think we have to deal with our own insecurities. Maybe I don't agree with that decision, maybe the doctor doesn't. But it's the patient's; it's his life. Who has more right?"

Now the question is, what should Ms. Winn do in *this* case when, let us suppose: (1) the patient, Mr. Saukin, genuinely does not want to be resuscitated; and (2) Dr. Cunningham, after finally discussing the matter with her, agrees that the law should be changed to permit "no codes"—at least when requested by patients like Mr. Saukin—but that until such changes are made he sees no alternative to responding to all such patients with full codes? On the one hand, Ms. Winn believes that she is morally required to respect Mr. Saukin's wishes and that her moral views on the matter are well-grounded and shared by many others, including the patient and Dr. Cunningham. On the other hand, what many regard as antiquated laws and Dr. Cunningham's concern for the letter of the law require her to override Mr. Saukin's wishes by carrying out a full code.

Ms. Winn knows that some nurses pretend to follow the law by carrying out "slow codes." That is, when a patient who is in a situation similar to that of Mr. Saukin arrests, some nurses take the defibrillator into the room slowly and fumble getting the airway in place; but in the end, as they know they must, they do the full code. The patients survive sometimes; but, according to Ms. Winn, "only to spend a few more days in agony before finally dying." However, Ms. Winn does not want to compromise herself and carry out a slow code under the guise of a full one.

In deciding whether to conscientiously refuse to comply with the orders for a full code, Ms. Winn needs to explore her reasoning with other people— other nurses, her nursing supervisors, Mr. Saukin and his family, and Dr. Cunningham if possible. Thoughtful discussion with others will not only help insure that she has not overlooked certain important considerations; it may also change the views of others and possibly soften or eliminate Ms. Winn's dilemma. Above all, if she decides that she simply cannot participate in a full code, she must be sure that arrangements are made to insure that her participation is not indispensable to carry out a full code. Finally, she must realize that conscientious refusal carries risks, which range from simply antagonizing others to reprimands or possibly even the loss of employment. For, as the examples of Arthur Miller, Winthrop Rockefeller, and Michael Heck, cited above, indicate, the price of personal integrity in a complex world is often extremely high. (For a discussion of the extent to which nurses ought to be involved in furthering legislative change in this and other areas, see Chapter 6.)

4. Nurse autonomy

In the following case, a nurse's autonomous actions resulted in a nurse-physician conflict.

4.7 Giving information to clients

Mrs. Tuma, a junior-college nursing instructor, requested that she be assigned to care for Mrs. W., a fifty-nine-year-old woman acutely ill with myelogenous leukemia, so that one of her nursing students could learn about chemotherapy. When the physician told Mrs. W. that she was dying and that the only hope for prolonging her life was chemotherapy, he described the painful and disfiguring side-effects of the treatment as well as the possibility of doing nothing. Although Mrs. W. had some degree of mental impairment caused by her condition, the physician believed that she was rational when he obtained both her and her family's consent for chemotherapy.

As Mrs. Tuma prepared the first chemotherapy dose, her student reported that she had found Mrs. W. crying. When Mrs. Tuma tried to comfort Mrs. W., Mrs. W. explained that she had fought leukemia for twelve years with God's help, by faithfully practicing the Mormon religion, by eating natural foods, and by avoiding drugs and stimulants. At this point Mrs. Tuma responded by discussing natural remedies for cancer with Mrs. W. She also determined, however, that Mrs. W. still consented to the chemotherapy and consequently initiated the chemotherapy intravenously as ordered. But Mrs. W. pleaded with Mrs. Tuma to return in the evening to discuss various natural treatments with her son and daughter-in-law.

When the daughter-in-law learned of the scheduled evening meeting with Mrs. Tuma, she phoned the doctor, who told her to attend the meeting and get the nurse's name. Early in the evening, the doctor phoned an order to suspend the chemotherapy because of Mrs. W.'s changed attitude. After Mrs. Tuma's discussion with the family, which included chemotherapy and its side-effects, alternatives provided by natural foods and herbs, the unavailability of Laetrile in the United States, and Mrs. W.'s problem of obtaining blood transfusions if she were to terminate chemotherapy, all agreed that Mrs. W.'s best course was to continue with chemotherapy.

Later in the evening the physician ordered the chemotherapy to be resumed. The next day he demanded that the college remove Mrs. Tuma from her position, which the college authorities consequently did. He also complained to the hospital, which notified the State Board of Nurses, which, in turn, initiated a petition for the suspension or revocation of Mrs. Tuma's license. The State Board Hearing Officer determined that Mrs. Tuma had interfered with the physician-patient relationship, an act that constituted unprofessional conduct; and the Board suspended her license for six months. Mrs. W. died two weeks after the chemotherapy was started.[33]

An examination of this case reveals arguments that support as well as some that oppose Mrs. Tuma's actions. A nurse, *as a person*, has the right to function autonomously as does every other person. Every person—client, physician, or nurse—can demand that he or she be recognized *as a person* worthy of dignity and respect with the right to act autonomously and to make justifiable claims on others for these general rights. However, the physician did not lodge a complaint against her as a person. Rather, in her discussions with Mrs. W., Mrs. Tuma had acted *as a nurse*. As Sister A. Teresa Stanley pointed out in her discussion of this case, no ethical dilemma would have resulted had a neighbor discussed the same information with Mrs. W.[34]

Yet Mrs. W.'s questions about alternative treatments made a claim upon Mrs. Tuma for information; and Mrs. Tuma agreed since she believed that she, as a nurse, should meet Mrs. W.'s needs. Both Mrs. Tuma and Mrs. W. perceived Mrs. Tuma's role as that of a well-informed care provider, someone who knew about and could explain alternative cancer treatments. Further, the professional nursing role, as Mrs. Tuma understood it, allowed her to insure that a client's consent to therapy was fully informed.[35] As Sally Gadow explained in a discussion of existential advocacy, "Patients can be assisted in reaching decisions which express their complex totality as individuals only by nurses who themselves act out of the same explicit self-unity, allowing no dimension of themselves to be exempt from the professional relation."[36] Acceptance of this notion, with its requirements for recognition of a nurse *as a person*, necessitates that a nurse be allowed to act autonomously in her nursing role.

Clearly, however, Mrs. Tuma had placed herself in a risky situation. Even though she included in her definition of the nursing role that nurses function autonomously, she recognized from the outset that not all persons, including the physician, shared that viewpoint.[37] In her state, the nursing role did not confer upon nurses the privilege of autonomous action in a situation such as that involving Mrs. W. The Hearing Officer for the Board of Nurse Examiners disallowed as evidence the American Nurses' Association Code for Nurses, because the Board had not adopted it, as well as any testimony or definitions by the ANA. He determined that Mrs. Tuma had interfered with the physician-patient relationship, which constituted unprofessional conduct. Thus, the Board judged that Mrs. Tuma did not have the privilege of functioning autonomously in her role as a nurse in this situation since her actions interfered with the physician-patient relationship.[38] To the Board, the nurse-client relationship apparently played a secondary role.[39]

A nurse in a situation similar to that of Mrs. Tuma could respond in a number of different ways. She could assume the traditional deferential role and do nothing autonomously. Or she could play an expert doctor-nurse game, pretend that she knew nothing when the client asked, and later, if possible, indirectly get the doctor to discuss alternative cancer treatments with the client. Or she could view the physician's presentation of only two choices (chemotherapy with its terrible side effects or no treatment) as unacceptable while at the same time recognizing that such a presentation of choices falls well within the acceptable scope of medical practice. Given this viewpoint, she could explain a variety of treatments during her initial contact with the patient, and later she could discuss the reasons for her actions with the physician. If, after she told the physician about a future family meeting, the physician ordered her not to proceed, the nurse could conscientiously refuse to follow the order and meet with the family as scheduled. If the physician filed a complaint, the State Board of Nurses might react as they did in the Tuma case. The physician might, however, have responded favorably at the outset if the nurse had clearly indicated that she was not challenging his special role with the patient but was acting as a professional who notified others of her intentions and shared her reasoning with them.

A nurse may also choose to act autonomously in a situation in which she knows her actions are not illegal but will lead, nevertheless, to unpleasantness for her. The following is such a case.

4.8 COPD team

JoAnne Kurtzman, head nurse of a fifty-bed acute care medical unit in which more than half of the patients have pulmonary problems, finds that pressures in her work come from doctors, staff, and the nursing and hospital administrations. To her, "other departments within the hospital have ideas of what they think nursing should be doing, and it is the nurse who is left to pull it all together." Her involvement in forming the COPD (chronic obstructive pulmonary disease) team represents such an attempt.

Mrs. Kurtzman described the situation: "We (the nursing staff) feel strongly that all departments should work closely together for the patient's benefit; and we thought one of the most effective ways to provide good care for our pulmonary patients would be through a team that includes nurses, respiratory therapists, and the Home Care Coordinator, who is a social worker. We were all to sit down once a week to make sure all the patients' needs were being met and to check that we were not each teaching the same thing to individual patients. We could all reinforce one another's teaching, and we would be aware of what each of us was doing.

"However, the COPD team is now viewed as a great threat. The physicians are totally against it and are slamming it. They feel that we are invading their territory. Doctors, such as Dr. Pickens, a pulmonary specialist, come along and say, 'No, you can't do this unless I order it.' Yet the Director of Nurses is very supportive and encourages us not to lower ourselves to the level at which some physicians used to see us performing; and the nursing staff knows that nursing is something in its own right and not just following through on medical orders.

"The doctors are showing they are against the COPD team effort by reprimanding nurses if an order is not carried out exactly the way they want it carried out. The other day Dr. Pickens ordered a nebulizer for a patient for bedside use. He came in the next morning and learned that the afternoon nurse had not gotten it. He demanded to know why, and I said it was my responsibility to look into it and that I would take care of it. That didn't

satisfy him. He got her phone number and demanded that she explain herself. She had worked late the night before, but he called her first thing in the morning for such a small item. The nurse told him, correctly, that the hospital happened to be out of them temporarily and would have one coming. I felt like Dr. Pickens was saying, 'You can't even carry out medical orders that I give you, so how could you even think about doing something on your own.'

"I find this attitude completely overwhelming. I think I should try to stay calm and composed, especially in front of my staff, since it would hurt the staff and patients if I were to create additional friction between doctors and nurses. I try to be the go-between and encourage the nurses' professionalism and their contribution to the doctor's overall plan of care for the patient. But I'm questioning how the COPD team can ever function."

What Mrs. Kurtzman may be asking is: "At what times, if any, should a nurse act autonomously without the approval or against the wishes of a physician?" A client's right to high-quality nursing care makes a claim upon nurses to provide such care. Mrs. Kurtzman and her staff believe that the COPD team provides better care than they could provide without it; therefore, they have a duty to make the team function.

The physicians in this situation do not view the nurses' activities as falling within the realm of nursing practice. Yet they seem to have no legal basis for complaint against the COPD team which, as Mrs. Kurtzman explained, does not expand the nurses' role but aims to facilitate better communication between professionals who work with individual patients. Lacking a legal basis for complaint, the physicians cannot expect the State Board of Nurses to control the nurses in their interest. Nor can they expect the Director of Nurses to help block the COPD team; she clearly supports independent, responsible nursing action. They can, however, make life difficult for the staff and the head nurse. When compared with legal and organizational pressures, unit-level unpleasantness is less threatening to a nurse's autonomous behavior. That the physicians must use petty inconveniences rather than legal or institutional pressures to block team functioning demonstrates the effectiveness of the nursing hierarchy's support of nursing practice.

The cases in this chapter raise the question, "At what times, if any, should a nurse act autonomously without the approval or against the wishes of a physician?" If her actions are based upon a client's just claim for her services, she is obligated to fulfill her duty to him or her. A nurse must recognize, however, when she acts autonomously, as a person, that her privilege to take that action, as a nurse, may be questioned and, at times, may lead to legal difficulties. Yet in certain special situations the nurse may choose to act autonomously, knowing full well that she is choosing to fulfill her moral obligations at the risk of legal prosecution. In many other cases in which her actions are clearly legal, she should recognize that she may have to tolerate much unpleasantness as the penalty for autonomous behavior.

5. Fixing responsibility

Much of nursing care occurs as part of team action that involves nurses and physicians as well as numerous other persons. The composition of various teams differs depending upon their functions, as, for example, an operating room team, a resuscitation team, a primary care team, a rehabilitation team, or a dialysis team. As Edmund Pellegrino has pointed out, the common feature of the health team is its collective action with final accountability belonging in one sense to each team member, and in another sense to the entire team.[40]

One difficulty in a transitory team, which comes together to provide services for an individual patient, and which disbands when that particular person leaves the institution, is in defining who is accountable for the care it provides.

4.9 Treatment of urinary tract infection

Mary Beth Mezinski had worked in various hospitals and nursing positions for nine years—as a nurse aide, ward clerk, nurse extern when a student nurse, graduate nurse for a short time, and staff nurse. She had applied recently for the position of in-service instructor for the ICU, Burn Unit, and Emergency Room nursing staffs in the large private hospital where she was employed.

Gladys Cary, admitted to Mary Beth's unit with a myocardial infarction, had been complaining constantly of irritation and painful urination. Two urine specimens had been sent to the laboratory and, on the third day, Mary Beth sent another which she described as "the pussiest urine upon catheterization I have ever seen." At that time, she called the intern, Dr. Bob McClintock, and told him about Mrs. Cary's urine and that the specimen was the third to be sent to the lab in three days.

The next morning Mary Beth learned that Mrs. Cary had not been started on any antibiotics. Nothing had been done about her problem, and she was urinating blood and mucus. When Dr. McClintock came on the floor with Dr. Valois, the internist whom he was following, Mary Beth, conscious that

Mrs. Cary was lying in pain while nothing was being done, was ready. As a nurse, Mary Beth knew that she "couldn't give Mrs. Cary quality care while she was so uncomfortable" with the urinary problem. Mary Beth also knew that she was being considered for the hospital's instructor position and that Dr. Valois was an old friend of the Director of Nursing who would soon decide the appointment. She did not want Dr. Valois to think she would be too critical and difficult to work with, and she knew her Director valued nurses who could get along well with the medical staff. But she also knew of herself that, "As I get older in the profession, I get bolder. I'm not as afraid to speak up to interns and residents and some physicians about the quality of care that I see being given."

Knowing what she had to do, Mary Beth said to the intern, "You're just the man I want to see. I told you about this urine specimen yesterday." She knew she was not being very tactful and had put him on the defensive, but she continued, "How come you haven't ordered anything?" He snapped, "Would you want to write the orders?" When Mary Beth said she probably could, she noticed that Dr. Valois walked away from them and wondered if he felt embarrassed by the argument. When Dr. McClintock said that the cultures were not back, Mary Beth retorted that they were and proceeded to enumerate the findings. To his excuse that he had not known, she countered that he could have telephoned the lab. At that, he grabbed the chart and said he would assess Mrs. Cary. Mary Beth followed the doctors into the room and back to the nurse's station, where they wrote a couple of orders. As they started to walk down the hall, she checked the orders and, to her frustration, found that nothing had been done about the urinary problem. She again asked them what they wanted to do about it. Dr. McClintock answered that he'd be back; and Mary Beth, still angry, muttered, "I'll expect you." He did return in half an hour and wrote some antibiotics orders, which were started immediately IV. But, as Mary Beth later said, "He was really hosed off at me, and I was really pissed off at him, and he knew it."

That afternoon Dr. McClintock came back and apologized for losing his temper. Mary Beth accepted his apology but told him that she "wasn't about to back down because I really felt that I was right in the situation." It struck her as unusual that three days later Dr. McClintock sat down with her and told her that she had really put Dr. Valois on the spot that day. For, not only had the intern failed to act immediately when called, but Dr. Valois had somehow missed the problem for three days. She admitted knowing that she might be criticizing Dr. Valois through her attack on an intern, but she had felt that something had to be done. Dr. McClintock agreed that she had been tenacious. Dr. Valois never said anything about the incident to her. A few

weeks later she received her new appointment. According to Mary Beth, she
and Dr. McClintock developed "a close working relationship."

This case raises questions relating to responsibility: "What should a nurse do when she disagrees with a physician's actions? Or if she thinks that a physician is following an unsafe practice? Who is responsible for monitoring individual and team competence? To whom are lapses reported—the person making the error, the team, the institution?"

A discussion of these questions must include both individual and team responsibilities. "Personal" physicians admit their patients to a hospital, and a patient quickly enters a relationship with the hospital (through a team composed of the personal physician, resident physicians, consulting physicians, nurses, therapists, and social workers) which is very much like the relationship a patient has with his own physician. A patient's right to effective medical treatment obligates his or her physician to provide that treatment. When a patient is admitted to a hospital, he or she makes a similar claim upon the hospital for safe, effective, morally responsible care, which the hospital fulfills through the employment of health care workers, including nurses. According to Pellegrino's view, one can interpret the responsibilities of a health team in two ways. In one way, responsibility is allocated only to individuals. In the other, responsibility is allocated to the team and is not reducible to individuals solely.

According to the interpretation of team ethics that allocates responsibility only to individuals, Pellegrino suggested that the problem of monitoring, correcting and revealing a fellow team member's incompetence is an unavoidable complication. Unfortunately, when some member fails to perform competently, his or her failure blocks or compromises the actions of other team members.[41] In Case 4.9, the physician's failure to treat Mrs. Cary for her urinary tract infection seriously compromised Mary Beth's attempts to provide high-quality nursing care. Therefore, Mary Beth's duty to provide nursing care obligated her to act in a way which would make certain the competent functioning of other team members; thus, in order to meet her own professional obligations, Mary Beth had to convince the physicians to assess Mrs. Cary's need for treatment of the urinary infection.

Furthermore, according to the interpretation of the team ethic that allocates responsibility to the entire team, all team members are accountable for the patient's well-being. Therefore, in this situation, all were to blame when the team's total care (which included overlooking signs of infection) resulted in Mrs. Cary's discomfort. In situations in which lapses in competence recur or bring discomfort or danger to a patient or in which optimal care is not given, the entire team may be morally (and legally) culpable.[42]

Mary Beth had two reasons for convincing the physicians to assess Mrs. Cary more thoroughly: First, as an individual professional, she was directly obligated to give the best possible nursing care, but the physicians' lapse of competence compromised her efforts. Second, she was obligated as a team member for Mrs. Cary's total care, which was frustrated by the physicians' lapse of competence. Given these reasons, Mary Beth was obligated to obtain optimum medical care for Mrs. Cary, which answers the first two questions the case raised. The actions a nurse should take, when she disagrees with a physician's actions or when she thinks that a physician is following an unsafe practice, must be based upon her responsibilities to the client both in her capacities as an individual practitioner and as a team member. The nurse may develop several strategies to meet her responsibilities. Mary Beth chose not to play a doctor-nurse game; after alerting Dr. McClintock, taking independent steps to have the laboratory results available, and waiting for the physicians to act, she chose to confront Dr. McClintock directly about his inaction. Evidently, her intense commitment to Mrs. Cary's welfare and the seriousness of the situation mitigated any real or imagined errors in etiquette that she may have made, and she and Dr. McClintock were able later to work well together. Although Mary Beth cannot *justify* the intemperate way in which she conveyed her objections, her conduct under the circumstances is in our view *excusable*.[43]

The answer to the third question, "Who is responsible for monitoring individual and team competence?" is based on the same dual interpretation of responsibility. Since each professional is responsible for his or her own actions, and since as a team member each professional is also responsible for the team's total effectiveness, each member of the team is obligated to monitor both the activities that affect his or her services and the outcome of the team's efforts. Of course, all team members cannot be aware of all aspects of one another's activities. Each professional, however, will be able to assess to varying degrees the effectiveness of other team members since the whole team focuses its attention on the same client.

Difficulty arises in answering the last question, "To whom are lapses reported?" The dual interpretation of responsibility suggests that insofar as responsibility can be allocated to an individual, that individual is also responsible for correcting his or her error. But to correct a problem an individual needs to learn of it.

Given the power structure of the health professions, some persons—

perhaps especially physicians—often view themselves as more important than other members of their health care team. Open communication in such situations is sometimes difficult. Ideally, the nurse should talk directly to the person whom she believes to have made an error, but telling another person about a suspected lapse of competence is a delicate matter. When the nurse cannot trace the problem to an individual, she should share the information with the whole team. Within the health team structure, the most effective course of action is usually for the nurse to report any lapse of competence to the person or persons who are directly responsible and to involve other people in the nursing and medical hierarchy only after attempting to solve the problem at its source.

Notes

1. George Rosen, *From Medical Police to Social Medicine: Essays on the History of Health Care* (New York: Science History Publications, 1974), p. 296.
2. Catherine P. Murphy, "The Moral Situation in Nursing," in Elsie L. Bandman and Bertram Bandman, *Bioethics and Human Rights* (Boston: Little, Brown), p. 315.
3. Joann Ashley, *Hospitals, Paternalism, and the Role of the Nurse* (New York: Columbia University, Teachers College Press, 1976), pp. 8-15.
4. Beatrice J. Kalisch and Philip A. Kalisch, "An Analysis of the Sources of Physician-Nurse Conflict," 7 *Journal of Nursing Administration* (January, 1977): 52.
5. Marjorie J. Stenberg, "The Search for a Conceptual Framework as a Philosophic Basis for Nursing Ethics: An Examination of Code, Contract, Context, and Covenant," *Military Medicine* (January, 1979): 13.
6. Kalisch and Kalisch, "An Analysis of the Sources of Physician-Nurse Conflict," 51-52.
7. Murphy, "The Moral Situation in Nursing," p. 315.
8. Leonard Stein, "The Doctor-Nurse Game," *American Journal of Nursing* 68 (January, 1968): 101-105.
9. Health Law Center and Charles J. Streiff, eds., *Nursing and the Law,* 2d ed. (Rockville, Maryland: Aspen Systems Corporation, 1975), p. 51.
10. Lucie Young Kelly, *Dimensions of Professional Nursing*, 3rd ed. (New York: Macmillan, 1975), pp. 122-24.
11. Bonnie Bullough, "The Law and the Expanding Nursing Role," *American Journal of Public Health* 66 (March 1976): 249-54; Darlene M. Trandel-Korenchuck and Keith M. Trandel-Korenchuck, "How State Laws Recognize Advanced Nursing Practice," *Nursing Outlook* 26 (November, 1978): 713-19.
12. Barbara Ehrenreich, "The Health Care Industry: A Theory of Industrial Medicine," *Social Policy* 6 (November/December, 1975): 7.
13. Kalisch and Kalisch, "An Analysis of the Sources of Physician-Nurse Conflict," 53.

14. Kelly, *Dimensions of Professional Nursing,* p. 169.
15. American Nurses' Association, *Facts about Nursing 76-77* (Kansas City, Missouri: American Nurses' Association, 1977), p. 4; David T. Abalos, "Strategies of Transformation in the Health Delivery System," *Nursing Forum* 17 (1978): 306.
16. Marlene Kramer, *Reality Shock: Why Nurses Leave Nursing* (St. Louis: C. V. Mosby, 1974), p. 21.
17. Carol A. Garant, "The Process of Effecting Change in Nursing," *Nursing Forum* 17 (1978): 158.
18. Loretta C. Ford, "A Nurse for All Settings: The Nurse Practitioner," *Nursing Outlook* 27 (August, 1979): 519.
19. Mary Gamer, "The Ideology of Professionalism," *Nursing Outlook* 27 (February, 1979): 110; See also Barbara Ehrenreich, "The Purview of Political Action," in *The Emergence of Nursing as a Political Force* (New York: National League for Nursing, 1979), pp. 11-17.
20. Bonnie Moore Randolph and Clydene Ross-Valliere, "Consciousness Raising Groups," *American Journal of Nursing* 79 (May, 1979): 922-24.
21. See Dorothea F. Orem, *Nursing: Concepts of Practice* (New York: McGraw-Hill, 1971), pp. 47-50, 115.
22. From a case collected by Leah L. Curtin, Acting Director, National Center for Nursing Ethics, Cincinnati, Ohio. It is one of sixty documented cases collected by NCNE.
23. Not only what a nurse says but the way in which she says it is important. While not advocating continuation of the doctor-nurse game, the authors recognize the need for nurses to be highly skillful in talking with certain physicians, especially those who cling to outmoded or stereotypical views of nursing.
24. In the actual situation, Ms. Pulec did choose to ask a third resident who, after listening to her reasons, told her that she was correct and cancelled the feedings order.
25. John Rawls, *A Theory of Justice* (Cambridge, Mass.: Harvard University Press, 1971), pp. 368-71.
26. This fictitious case was prepared especially for this volume. For a recent discussion of the unprecedented issues it raises see the series of responses accompanying John Fletcher, "Ethics and Amniocentesis for Fetal Sex Identification," *Hastings Center Report,* 10 (February, 1980): 15-20.
27. James F. Childress, "Appeals to Conscience," *Ethics* 89 (1978-1979): 316-17.
28. Bernard Williams, "A Critique of Utilitarianism," in J. J. C. Smart and Bernard Williams, *Utilitarianism For and Against* (Cambridge: Cambridge University Press, 1973), pp. 115-17.
29. Childress, "Appeals to Conscience," pp. 318-21.
30. Herbert Fingarette, *Self-Deception* (London: Routledge and Kegan Paul, 1969), *passim* and especially pp. 138-39.
31. Robert M. Veatch, *Death, Dying, and the Biological Revolution: Our Last Quest for Responsibility* (New Haven: Yale University Press, 1976), pp. 116-63; David L. Jackson and Stuart Youngner, "Patient Autonomy and 'Death with Dignity,'" *New England Journal of Medicine* 301 (August 23, 1979): 404-408.

32. See Robert M. Veatch, "Death and Dying: The Legislative Options," *Hastings Center Report* 7 (October, 1977): 5–8.
33. Based on a case described by Sister A. Teresa Stanley, "Is It Ethical to Give Hope to a Dying Person?" *Nursing Clinics of North America* 14 (March, 1979): 69–71.
34. *Ibid.*, 75.
35. Jolene L. Tuma, "Professional Misconduct," (Letter) *Nursing Outlook* 25 (September, 1977): 546.
36. Sally Gadow, "Existential Advocacy: Philosophical Foundation of Nursing," presented to the Four State Consortium on Nursing and the Humanities at its Phase I Conference, "Nursing and the Humanities: A Public Dialogue," Farmington, Connecticut, November 11, 1977, pp. 16–17.
37. Stanley, "Is It Ethical to Give Hope to a Dying Person," 78.
38. *Ibid.*, 75–76.
39. Three years after Mrs. Tuma's license was suspended, she won a reversal of the suspension ruling when the state's supreme court made a unanimous decision in her favor. Although now licensed, she is not in practice because she "feels it is unwise" given the climate of her local medical-nursing community. The junior college has not reinstated her. "Nurse Upheld in Idaho Court Case," *Concern for Dying* 5 (Fall, 1979): 7.
40. Edmund D. Pellegrino, "The Ethics of Team Care: Some Notes on the Morality of Collective Decision Making," presented to the American Cancer Society, Second National Conference on Cancer Nursing, St. Louis, Missouri, May 9, 1977, p. 6.
41. *Ibid.*, pp. 7–8.
42. *Ibid.*, p. 9.
43. The notion of an act that is excusable, though not justifiable, is important in a wide variety of contexts in ethics and the law. People who violate laws or moral principles under conditions of duress may be excused for what they do, even though their actions cannot, strictly speaking, be justified. A harried parent, for example, who loses his or her temper and yells at or even spanks a persistently cranky or annoying child, may be excused for what he or she does even though it cannot be justified. So too, if a nurse "loses her cool" after reasonable attempts to correct a situation have been unsuccessful, an exasperated outburst, though perhaps not justified and even counterproductive, may under the circumstances be excused.

5

Ethical Dilemmas Among Nurses

1. Tensions between nurses

In their practice, nurses work closely with other nurses. Since a nurse's activities normally overlap with those of other nurses, her practice affects and is affected by the practice of others. In addition, most nurses either supervise or are supervised by nurses. Given such interdependence, ethical dilemmas involving relationships among nurses are inevitable and understandable. The following case illustrates one such dilemma.

5.1 Medication cover-up

Jane Robinson, a twenty-eight-year-old nurse with a B.S.N. and several years nursing experience, has been working part time for three weeks in a small rural community hospital. She is evening charge nurse on a twenty-bed medical and pediatric floor two evenings a week and on a surgical floor the third evening. When Jane accepted her position, she realized that she would be meeting a new set of challenges nearly every evening. One busy evening when a patient on the medical floor was supposed to get phenobarb, gr ¼, Jane mistakenly went to the wrong cabinet, took out codeine, gr ¼, and gave it to the patient. At the end of the shift Jane checked the narcotics count with Shirley Tucker, a thirty-two-year-old midnight LPN known for her thoroughness, who is planning to return to school to become an RN. As Shirley counted aloud the remaining narcotics and barbiturates, Jane wrote the same total that had previously been noted for each rather than writing the actual count. She did not realize what she had done.

The next night Shirley brought the matter of the extra phenobarb and the missing codeine to Jane's attention, told Jane that she had "goofed," and said that she had fixed Jane's error during the night. She had "jimmied" the books by throwing away a phenobarb and by falsely writing in the codeine book that she had given codeine, gr ¼, to a patient who conveniently had an order for it. The patient to whom Jane had mistakenly given the codeine apparently had had no side effects and had been discharged during the day.

Jane does not know if she should report her mistake. On the one hand, she thinks she can overlook her medication error since the patient was not harmed and, although Shirley knows of the mistake, it is doubtful that others will discover it. By not reporting her error to the nursing administration, Jane could keep her total number of incident reports at a low level. She knows that many nurses in the hospital believe that other nurses interpret a low number of incident reports as "no error" nursing which, they believe, is synonymous with "good" nursing. Therefore, some nurses tend not to report small errors. On the other hand, Jane could easily make an incident report. She knows that as an honest person she ought to report her error, and she believes that honesty is an important part of her professional identity. Further, she believes that she should follow hospital policy and rules. But in admitting her mistake, she would expose Shirley's cover-up activities, including the falsification of narcotics records.

Among the questions this case raises are: "To what extent, if any, should a nurse jeopardize her own or another's professional position by admitting an error, and must a nurse report a 'cover-up' in order to maintain her authority as an RN and effectiveness as a role model?"

Some basic information about relationships among nurses is necessary for a discussion of this case. Various general factors, as discussed in the previous chapter with regard to conflicts between nurses and physicians, also affect relationships between nurses. These include: remnants of the historical legacy of nursing; technological and social changes; the expanding scope of nursing practice; and the ideology of professionalism and the increased importance of education, especially with regard to baccalaureate and graduate degrees in nursing. We can see the effect of these factors on tensions in nursing relationships by examining personal variables among nurses and structural variables in nursing practice. Since both personal and structural variables tend to block and confuse efforts to engage in ethical inquiry, it is important to recognize them.

A. Personal variables among nurses

Nurses differ from one another in many ways. Nursing is traditionally a woman's profession, but not all nurses are women. Some men have been and are nurses, even though as early as 1880 women nurses outnumbered men eleven to one and at present outnumber them seventy to one.[1] Like male nurses, ethnic minority nurses are fewer in number than their comparative percentages in the general population. Desegregation of nursing schools did not begin until after World War II, and by 1951 only 3 percent of nursing students were black. At present some schools actively recruit minority students.[2] Sex and racial differences affect nursing relationships as they do relationships in other professions and in society generally. As the following discussion indicates, personal variables that add to tension in nursing relationships include a nurse's educational background, experience, view of nursing, and career goals.

All persons seeking to become registered nurses (RN) currently take the same licensure examination even though they may have graduated from one of three different educational programs—two-year associate degree, three-year hospital-based diploma, or four-year college or university baccalaureate program. Disagreement exists within the profession as to which program leads to "professional" and which to "technical" nursing since all three programs now lead to the same license—registered nurse. Persons seeking to become licensed practical or vocational nurses (LPN or LVN) study for approximately one year before taking a licensure examination for practical nurses.

Another personal variable is experience in nursing practice. We have seen that in certain circumstances an experienced and skillful nurse may have knowledge that an inexperienced physician lacks. So too, certain situations will arise in which an experienced nurse who has kept up with new developments and has changed her nursing practice accordingly may know more about a particular nursing problem than a recent graduate from a prestigious nursing program. The quality and usefulness of nursing experience, like other personal variables, differs among individual nurses.

Given the variety of their educational backgrounds and their varying nursing experiences, nurses understandably vary in their views of nursing. As previously discussed (see Chapter 4, Section 1), nurses not only provide bedside nursing care, but they give physical examinations, do health care teaching, etc. Common to nursing, however, is a shared legacy of belief as to what nursing is. Nurse-writers of the past and nurse-theorists of today stress that: (1) nursing assists both well and sick persons; (2) "health" is a general nursing goal; and (3) to accomplish the goal, nursing encompasses a wide range of activities based upon a problem-solving process that includes assessment, diagnosis, intervention, and evaluation.[3] Nurses, although they share a general historical view of nursing, place differing degrees of importance on various theoretical models of nursing and on various activities involved in the nursing process.

A nurse's career goal is also an important variable that sometimes increases tension in nursing relationships. Some nurses pursue nursing as a lifetime career, while others prefer not to work full time, especially during their child-rearing years. As Vern and Bonnie Bullough have pointed out, nursing leaders are generally those who are most able to devote time and energy to nursing; thus, it is no surprise that many nursing leaders are unmarried.[4] A number of changes such as the women's movement, tax credits for child care, and higher salaries could result in an increased number of married nurses becoming more active in the profession. But a gulf presently exists between general-duty nurses and nursing leaders. It is symptomatic that only 21 percent of the currently employed registered nurses belong to the American Nurses' Association; this suggests a low interest in professional organization among the rank and file.

To return to Case 5.1, notice that the educational background and experiences of the two persons involved are quite dissimilar; one is an RN with a B.S.N. and the other an LPN. They may or may not hold similar views of nursing or similar career goals. Note, however, that their responsibilities are the same regarding the end-of-shift narcotic and barbiturate count. In at least some respects they have been employed to carry out the same duties. The dilemma of the medication cover-up is made complex not only because of the personal variables involved but because of an equally important reason—the structure of nursing practice.

B. Structural variables in nursing practice

The structure of nursing practice varies according to the settings and staff assignment designs in which nurses practice. For most nurses, over 75 percent, the setting is a hospital.[5] Settings here include, for example, intensive care units, premature nurseries, medical inpatient care units, surgical inpatient care units, pediatric units, oncology units, inservice education programs, ambulatory care units, and obstetrical units. For other nurses the setting is an extended care facility. Still others are in clinics or the community, including, for example, offices, schools, and clients' homes.[6] For a few nurse practitioners the setting is independent practice.

In addition to the practice setting, a nurse's employer describes his or her job responsibilities and assignments. Institutions use the following basic designs for describing nursing staff assignments: case, functional, team, and primary care nursing or some variation or combination of these designs. In case nursing, a design followed especially in the 1920s, the head nurse assigns the total care of each patient to one nurse. According to the functional method, the head nurse assigns staff members specific tasks—as medication nurse, treatment nurse, bedside care nurse, etc. In team nursing, developed in the 1950s, a registered nurse team leader assigns duties to each team member, plans and coordinates care, serves as a resource person, and sometimes provides direct patient care. In primary care nursing, developed in the 1970s, a primary nurse accepts responsibility for the total twenty-four-hour care of a client by interviewing the client on admission, making a nursing diagnosis, issuing orders, and coordinating client activities with the client's physicians and family and with other health workers. Another staff nurse, termed an associate, cares for the client when the primary nurse is off duty, although the associate may phone the primary nurse to seek a change in nursing orders. Institutions that use the primary care design generally restructure the traditional positions of staff nurse, head nurse, and nurse administrator in order to include nurse clinical coordinators and nurse clinicians.[7]

Various writers have noted that nursing staff assignments, especially in institutional settings, have tended to ignore personal variables among nurses. Helen Burnside concluded that "regardless of the fact that nurses are taught that major differences exist between types of nurse practitioners, in most institutional settings nurses continue to perform similar tasks and assume nearly identical responsibilities along the entire continuum from practical nurses to baccalaureate graduates."[8] Salary and wage levels reflect this lack of differentiation. Starting institutional salaries for various types of nursing personnel, from LPNs to baccalaureate nurses, do not differ substantially in spite of differences in length and levels of training.[9] It is noteworthy, however, that change is occurring in the role of nurses. Myrtle Aydelotte has pointed out that nursing practice has become clinically focused and that the new trend in primary nursing care staffing assignments uses two distinct levels of nursing practitioners, professional and technical.[10] Specialization and stratification are increasing, but presently structural variables in nursing practice, combined with personal variables among nurses, tend to complicate and add significant tension to nursing relationships. Therefore, in analyzing ethical dilemmas that are primarily disagreements between nurses, it is important to recognize the extent to which these variables underlie the issues.

To return to "Medication cover-up," we can see similarities in the structural variables in that the RN and the LPN share the same rural hospital
setting and some of the same job responsibilities. In addition, since they do
not work the same shift, it is reasonable to assume that Jane, the RN, does
not supervise Shirley, the LPN, as often occurs in a traditional nursing
service hierarchy, but that they relate to one another more or less on an
equal basis. In terms of personal variables, however, differentiation appears.
The LPN's actions were based, at least in part, on the assumption that she
and Jane, the RN, shared the same view of nursing errors—the need to
minimize the number of small errors and to cover them up. Jane's concern
about how she should respond indicates that she does not unequivocally
share Shirley's viewpoint. But while it is reasonable to assume that personal
variables influence Jane's and Shirley's perception of the situation and of
one another, none of the variables changes the fact that their employer,
clients, and other health care providers expect that both women will provide
safe, effective, and responsible care. Further, nursing organizations have
adopted codes of ethics to guide their conduct. For example, the Code of
Ethics of the National Federation of Licensed Practical Nurses states that
LPNs must "recognize and have a commitment to meet the ethical, moral,
and legal obligations to the practice of practical/vocational nursing." As
Carmen Ross points out in her discussion of this code, examples of unethical
procedures would be deliberate misuse of narcotics and barbiturates and
falsely charting procedures and observations.[11] The Code for Nurses adopted
by the American Nurses' Association states that "The nurse acts to safeguard the client and the public when health care and safety are affected
by [the] incompetent, unethical, or illegal practice of any person." The
ANA's interpretive statements of the code underscore the nurse's primary
commitment to the client, direct her to express concern to any person
engaging in a questionable practice and to report to the responsible administrative person when a client's welfare is threatened. In terms of accountability,
Jane and Shirley are responsible for their own acts.

In complicated cases, a number of different factors affect the situation.
Therefore, in order to take a position on Case 5.1, we will make the
following assumptions:

1. The client who received the wrong medication needs no treatment to
   counteract the effects of the error.
2. Jane, the RN, wants to behave in a forthright, honest fashion in all her
   dealings, private and professional.
3. Little chance exists that if Jane reports her error a change to a more

nearly error-free system of medication preparation, administration, and recording will result.

4. Shirley's, the LPN's, reasons for covering up Jane's error were grounded in good intentions—to give Jane, a new employee, the benefit of the doubt in terms of number of errors and to protect her from criticism for having too many errors. Yet her intentions, however good they may have been, have no bearing on our judgment that throwing away a barbiturate and falsifying records are wrong. Thus, while Shirley may not be a bad person, she acted wrongly in this situation.

5. While Shirley did not harm any clients, and the cost of the wasted phenobarbital was negligible, her waste of materials and falsification of records, if carried on over time and in other situations, could result in harm to clients.

6. Simply reporting Shirley's cover-up would probably result in a poor working relationship among Jane, Shirley, and other nurses who have worked with Shirley; and it may result in strong disciplinary action against Shirley, thus creating a situation that could block provision of good nursing care and could possibly cause the removal of an otherwise effective LPN.

7. If Jane chooses to take no action concerning the cover-up, she is condoning Shirley's activities and, thus, making herself partly responsible for the cover-up and harmful consequences that may arise in the future.

8. Since Shirley enjoys a reputation as a thorough worker and aims to become a registered nurse, she probably is motivated to function in a manner acceptable to a nurse like Jane.

Given the first three assumptions, if Jane should decide to report her error, it would be not to prevent harm to the client but rather to maintain a conception of herself as an honest professional. Given Shirley's involvement and assumptions (4) and (5), Jane must decide whether Shirley's motivation to be helpful to Jane cancels out the wrong she actually did. Notice, however, that had Shirley's action resulted in harm, excusing her behavior would not be possible. Given the last three assumptions, Jane must take some action if she is to maintain an independent identity as a responsible person and a professional nurse even though her actions would carry risk for Shirley, herself, and, if nursing care is affected, their clients. Finally, although Jane is not Shirley's supervisor, Shirley would probably try to act in accord with her suggestions.

We think that Shirley's reasons for her wrongful acts, the fact that the acts were not harmful even though wrong, and the possible deterioration of good

nursing care and/or removal of the LPN, override Jane's prima facie obligation to report Shirley's conduct. Thus, Jane should talk with Shirley and
explain that while she recognizes Shirley's friendly motive for the cover-up,
she also recognizes that such acts are wrong. She should explain that
although in this situation no harm resulted, the probability that harm could
result requires Shirley to refrain absolutely from such acts. Further, she
should tell Shirley that, although she expects no more false reporting, if it
occurs, she will report it to their supervisor.

The questions this case raised initially were: "To what extent, if any,
should a nurse jeopardize her own or another's professional position by
admitting an error; and, must a nurse report a 'cover-up' in order to maintain
her authority as an RN and her effectiveness as a role model?" Our analysis,
while not directly answering these questions, illustrates that there may be
situations in which, all things considered, the best course of action lies
somewhere between two extremes when neither is fully satisfactory and each
has something to recommend it. In this case, simply reporting the error
shows too little concern for the LPN's good intentions, and simply ignoring
the situation sets a dangerous precedent.

2. Respect for persons

Underlying the previous discussion, with its emphasis upon the nurse's
decision about what she ought to do, is a presumption that the nurse is a self-
determining person. A person can not be held responsible for the consequences of her actions unless she is allowed to judge and choose for herself.
Respect for persons, a principle discussed in Chapter 3, Section 2, and which
we will explore in the following case, involves acknowledging people's rights
as persons to do as they see fit within certain limits.[12]

5.2 Judgmental comments

*Last week, public health nurse Mary Ann Rhoads went to a hospital to visit
one of her clients, Debra Sharpe, who had just had her second baby.
According to Mary Ann, "Debra is a seventeen-year-old uneducated black
person from the South so it's very difficult for me to understand her thick
dialect. I went to the nursery to see the baby, and one of the nurses looked
disgustedly at me and asked, 'How old is that mother, anyway?' I said,
'Seventeen,' and she sneered, 'I thought so.' I felt that she was placing a very
negative judgment on Debra and her baby."*

Mary Ann did not say anything to the nurse, but now she is bothered. "I realize I have some health values. I know that Debra's baby is going to be a high-risk child; in fact, the older sibling had lead poisoning. But the decision to have this second baby was Debra's decision; my own values about her child's future health are irrelevant. All people make decisions about their lives for one reason or another. If we don't know what those decisions and reasons are, and even if we do, we can't pass judgment on another person."

Mary Ann does not know what to do. She thinks she has two problems. First, she does not know if she should return to the nursery and attempt to talk with the nurse. Is it appropriate for her, a nurse from one agency, to advise a nurse who is employed in another agency? Second, she does not know whether she should try to force her own values on another person, specifically, the nurse who made the judgmental comment.

Before examining Mary Ann's concern about her relationship with the nursery nurse, we need to discuss the two nurses' views of the young mother, Debra. Mary Ann thinks her own values about Debra's decision to have a second baby are irrelevant at this point and that she cannot pass judgment on others. The nursery nurse implied that Debra was wrong to have the baby.

Mary Ann's statements indicate that she accepts a principle of respect for persons which holds that, generally and with certain qualifications, each person is in the best position to determine what will satisfy her or his interest—i.e., each person is in the best position to determine her or his conception of the good and what means are most suitable to realizing it. According to this theory, a "person" is a being who is aware of herself or himself, not just as a process, happening, or thing, but as an agent, making decisions that make a difference to the way the world goes, and able to determine and attempt to realize some conception of the good.[13] *Respect for persons* involves acknowledging a person's right to pursue her or his conception of the good so long as doing so does not interfere with the right of other persons to do likewise. In terms of the principle of respect for persons, Mary Ann acknowledged Debra's right to decide to have another baby which, of course, would not interfere with the rights of others to have babies. Mary Ann treated Debra as a person since she did not interfere with Debra's choice to have a baby; that is, she responded in a fashion that respected Debra's decision by continuing to offer nursing care to her and her children and by refraining from passing judgment on her.

Although basically sound, Mary Ann's understanding of the principle of respect of persons is mistaken in one crucial respect. Mary Ann's recognition of Debra's personhood, which includes recognition of her self-determination, freedom, and dignity, does not mean that Mary Ann could not or should not engage Debra in discussions involving health risks to her children and other health-related topics. Rather, the opposite is true. Mary Ann's respect for Debra as a person is a reason to engage in health teaching and rational discussion about what Debra ought to do. Mary Ann, in holding to the principle of respect for persons, must, of course, take into account Debra's point of view; she must acknowledge Debra's prima facie claim to noninterference; and she must not use her special status as a nurse to impose her values on Debra.[14] Mary Ann is mistaken, however, in thinking that her health values are irrelevant. When Mary Ann engages Debra in health teaching, Debra may decide to adopt some of Mary Ann's health values and information in making her own decisions about the health of her children or herself. Further, since Debra's right to noninterference is a prima facie claim and not an absolute right, Mary Ann may override a particular decision of Debra's if she recognizes that it interferes with certain of the baby's rights. For example, a nurse might choose to override a mother's feeding plan if that plan would obviously lead to an infant becoming dangerously overweight. In short, although Mary Ann's respect for Debra as a person requires that she not resort to manipulation or coercion, it does allow and perhaps requires that she engage her in dialogue and, where she thinks Debra is misinformed, attempt to educate her or alter her views with rational persuasion. Mary Ann's mistake here is in part attributable to a failure to realize that Debra's right as a person to decide for herself what she will do with her life does not imply that all decisions made in this fashion are the right or best ones. (See Chapter 3, Section 3 for an account of the distinctions between rational persuasion, manipulation, and coercion.)

The nursery nurse's behavior and remarks to Mary Ann, on the other hand, probably indicate that she does not regard clients in the same way as Mary Ann. She may, like Mary Ann, believe in the importance of rights but believe that more important rights than Debra's are involved in the situation. For example, she may think that her right as a taxpayer to have lower taxes or to receive public services, which Debra's possible collection of public assistance would reduce to some extent, should override Debra's right to have a second baby. Or she may take a purely utilitarian view and believe that society's interest as a whole will be maximized if poor, uneducated, minority women like Debra are prevented from having a second child. Or she may simply be prejudiced and not have analyzed her feelings about Debra and her children.

Mary Ann's problems as she presented them in the case are, first, whether she should try to talk with the nursery nurse, an employee of another agency, and second, whether she should try to force her own values on another person. Both nurses should have as their primary concern the welfare of clients and, more specifically, Debra's and the baby's care. Mary Ann's worry about whether to discuss her concerns with the nursery nurse indicates that she views personal and/or structural variables as separating them as colleagues. Even though they may not be "peers," may not have equal standing in rank or class because of differences in educational background and other personal variables, and even though they differ in employment settings and nursing assignment responsibilities, both are equal as persons. As equal persons working to provide good nursing care to clients, each should be free to talk with the other about their practice of nursing; thus, Mary Ann should feel free to tell the hospital nurse about her concerns that focus on the primary issue in nursing—client care.

The second question, whether Mary Ann should try to force her values on another person, must be answered with a "no." This does not imply that she cannot try to engage the other in dialogue and use rational persuasion to convince her of the soundness of her values. On the contrary, dialogue with the nursery nurse, as opposed to manipulating, coercing or simply ignoring her is the way for Mary Ann to show respect for her as a person. If Mary Ann is to be consistent in her dealings with others, she has to respect the other nurse's right to formulate and express views, opinions, and actions just as she respects her client's right to do so. Therefore, she must deal with the nurse as a rational being. But the nurse, like Debra and all persons, has only a prima facie right to noninterference. Mary Ann could question the nurse's actions (prejudicial comments about a client) because she believes she can show that those actions could infringe upon a vulnerable client's basic rights of self-determination, freedom, and dignity. In this case, however, the nursery nurse's disgusted look and her sneered "I thought so," are heavily nonverbal and would be difficult to discuss meaningfully a week or more later.

In summary, Mary Ann is free to talk as a person and colleague with the nursery nurse. In accordance with the principle of respect for persons, she could engage the nurse in a rational discussion about poor young minority mothers and their rights as persons. In discussing respect for persons, she could point out that judgmental negative comments may undermine a client's dignity. The effect of such a discussion would depend upon the nursery nurse's ability and willingness to accept and use the information. Because so much time has elapsed since the incident, Mary Ann might well decide at this point not to revive the issue with the nurse. After thinking through this situation, however, she should now be prepared to deal with similar judgmental comments by nursing personnel as they occur.

3. Professional obligations

As we discussed in Chapter 4, Section 5, each nurse is responsible in one sense for her own professional practice and in another sense for the practice of the health care team of which she is a member. The following two cases present questions relating to a nurse's responsibility as a member, not of a health care team, but of the nursing profession.

5.3 Working extra hours

Diane MacIntyre has two and one-half years' experience as staff nurse on a general medical unit that serves many diabetic and stroke patients. As a team leader she both gives direct patient care and plans basic care for other nursing personnel to carry out. In the past, when she worked extra hours at home or in the hospital library writing procedures, the other nurses (especially another team leader, Arlene Estes, who is a single parent with three children) have said that Diane (who is single and without children) was foolish to work without pay. During the last few months Diane's attendance at weekly meetings of a multidisciplinary team composed of professionals from physical therapy, occupational therapy, and social services who are active in rehabilitation efforts on her floor, has strained her relationships with nursing coworkers. According to Diane, "The other nurses think I'm crazy to come in on my own time. I go to practically every weekly meeting, which are mainly on my days off. I get a lot of positive reinforcement from being with that group of people, and I think they have a little better impression of nursing due to my participation."

Diane's decision to participate with the multidisciplinary team stems from her desire to get more out of her job than just a paycheck and her conclusion that "nursing is one of those jobs that you really have to put a lot of effort into in order to get any satisfaction at all." She wants to show that "nursing is an important profession and nurses have something to contribute besides passing meds and giving baths." Despite her justification for working extra hours, Diane nevertheless feels hurt by the other nurses' reactions, especially those of her friend Arlene, whose skills and integrity she has always admired.

This case raises the following questions: "What are the obligations of being a member of the nursing profession? Do these obligations include attending meetings on one's own time and expense? Working overtime?" The American Nurses' Association Code for Nurses addresses the question of responsibility to the profession. Item 8 of the Code, which states that "The nurse participates in the profession's efforts to implement and improve standards of nursing," includes an interpretive statement that "The nurse has the responsibility to monitor these standards [ANA standards for nursing practice, service and education] in everyday practice and through *voluntary participation* [emphasis ours] in the profession's ongoing efforts to implement and improve standards at the national, state, and local levels." Item eleven, which states "The nurse collaborates with members of the health professions and other citizens in promoting community and national efforts to meet the health needs of the public," includes an interpretive statement that "The nurse should *actively seek to promote collaboration* [emphasis ours] needed for ensuring the quality of health services to all persons." The Code clearly expresses the view that nurses have obligations not only to themselves and to clients, but to the nursing profession as well. While not stating that participation in activities to improve nursing as a discipline may require extra working hours, the Code implies as much.

Very few nurses have established independent nursing practices; rather, agencies—hospitals, nursing homes, community health departments, schools, industries, physicians, health maintenance organizations, etc.—employ the vast majority of nurses. A nurse makes a contract with an agency in order to carry out her primary obligation to the client—the provision of safe, effective, responsible nursing, be it, in the words of the ANA Code, "the promotion of health, the prevention of illness," or "the alleviation of suffering." An employment contract, either written or oral, specifies a nurse's obligations in terms of working hours and specific responsibilities, as well as an agency's obligations in terms of pay, benefits, vacations, etc. In addition, nurses often feel obligated to do more than the contract specifies because they fall into the "compassion trap" by accepting the expectations of many agency employers, health care workers, and clients that nurses—members of a "helping profession"—will subordinate their own needs or desires to those of others.[15]

To return to the nurses in Case 5.3, both Diane and Arlene share high ideals about professionalism, and as dedicated nurses both are also affected by the "compassion trap," with its assumption that the nurse will sacrifice for others. Therefore, Diane is somewhat discouraged by Arlene's recent comments about only working for pay. Peggy Sayre, another nurse from a different unit in the hospital and a friend of both women, suggested that Diane, Arlene, and she talk during a break about problems relating to Diane's working extra. After listening to the other two nurses describe the situation, Peggy asked each of them why they felt as they did about working extra.

Diane had no difficulty in pointing out that her involvement with the interdisciplinary team and working on hospital procedures would lead to better care for a larger number of clients. She also emphasized that her professional goals of high-quality nursing care and the hospital's current inclusion of her in the multidisciplinary team were in perfect agreement.

Arlene acknowledged that Diane's contributions to client welfare were admirable but quickly shifted to her own feelings concerning Diane's extra work. Arlene believed that because Diane functioned as a "super nurse" the head nurse looked upon Arlene and several other nurses, who could not devote extra time to hospital matters, as less than adequate professional nurses. Further, they themselves were beginning to feel inadequate. One way for them to restore their private as well as professional self-esteem would be for them to match Diane's work load by working extra hours. Arlene predicted that client welfare would be negatively affected, however, since she and most of the other nurses would be worn out by the combination of home duties, regular job, and extra unpaid work.

Arlene also said that, perhaps more important, she believes the way a nurse feels about herself as a professional affects the way in which she approaches nursing care. Although Arlene did not think that her negative feelings about her current level of participation in nursing matters at the hospital had affected her practice, she thought that if her morale continued to deteriorate, her nursing might suffer. She also predicted that if the nurses continued to see themselves as inadequate, even though they did their best during every working hour, some of them would quit. The resulting nursing personnel turnover would cause confusion, and a reduction of the high-quality nursing care now being provided. Further, Arlene believed that if a high turnover rate persisted, the "good" that Diane's extra work did would be undermined.

Peggy thought that both Diane and Arlene had missed the major issue. As for Arlene, Peggy did not believe that the decline in unit morale and the increase in nursing staff turnover would be as great as Arlene predicted, but she agreed that these were important concerns. More important, she believed that Arlene, who recognized that she must meet her basic duties as a nurse and honor her contract with the hospital, had not completely accepted the view that idealized commitments to professional nursing might be overridden by other more stringent and immediate commitments, such as those to her children. To Peggy, Arlene, like all nurses, had personal as well as professional obligations; and Arlene, as a single parent, need not apologize for not working more than a forty-hour week. Peggy illustrated her point by describing a public health nurse, whom they all knew, who had been extremely active in collective-bargaining activities in the county health department. When her mother had become seriously ill and needed her every evening, the nurse could no longer attend special nightly meetings. Her obligations to her sick parent, while not excusing her from her contractual obligations to the health department, did excuse her from the additional commitments she had previously taken on. Arlene's personal obligations, like those of the public health nurse, were more basic and thus took precedence over her less stringent professional obligations.

Neither was Peggy convinced by Diane's argument that her professional nursing goals were being met, and that the end result would be an overall improvement in client welfare. Although she agreed with Diane that the initiation of a new program or change often required an initial period of voluntary effort, she argued that as soon as the program's value was recognized, it was necessary to press for its institutionalization. In Diane's case, Peggy believed, Diane had amply demonstrated the value of what she was doing. Therefore, she should now take steps to make hers a paying, institutionalized position. Peggy pointed out that since Diane's work depended entirely upon one nurse's willingness to work extra, when she left her current position for one with more responsibility—which all three nurses agreed that a young, effective nurse like Diane would do within a short time—there would probably be no one to carry on her good work. Nor, since the hospital had gotten Diane's work free, would their employer believe that another nurse would not also step forward to give free time and effort to the hospital.

Peggy predicted that at Diane's departure there would be no nursing contribution to the multidisciplinary team or to similar activities since no institutional changes to provide for participation by nurses would be made so long as Diane functioned as she did. Therefore, in the long run, clients would not be well served by nursing. Thus, Diane was not meeting her professional goals when the future was considered. Peggy summarized her position by saying that Diane's extra work was a problem because the nurses on the unit could not determine if Diane's special activities were merely an extension of her efforts to be professional by providing the highest quality nursing care possible or if she had slipped into the hospital's institutionalized system of devaluing nursing, although the system was obviously more subtle than that which nineteenth-century hospitals had used to exploit nurses.[16] To Peggy, the major issue was that if Diane continued to attend special meetings without compensation, she would actually support the notion that her activities were not truly part of a nurse's employee role and that the hospital had no obligation to support nurses who work long hours to write procedures and attend multidisciplinary team meetings.

To return to the questions raised by this case, a nurse has certain obligations to the nursing profession, as discussed in the ANA Code for Nurses. At times those obligations may include working overtime and attending meetings on one's own time and expense. But as this case illustrates, when a nurse critically examines her obligations, she may see that basic personal commitments sometimes override less stringent professional commitments that might be met by "working extra." She may also see that "working extra," while appearing to fulfill professional obligations and the ideal of compassionate service, may only superficially meet obligations to clients and may actually lead to a less desirable state of affairs not only for nursing colleagues and the nursing profession, but ultimately for clients.

In the following case, a nurse faces a somewhat different ethical dilemma than that involved in the problem of working extra hours. The questions the case raises involve conflict between a nurse's obligations as a nursing administrator and her desire to be helpful to her subordinate.

5.4 A nurse with a drug problem

Ms. Maria Romero, Associate Director of Nursing, is responsible for the daily nursing division operations of a three-hundred-bed-hospital. During the past year she has met several times with Pam Altmann, a staff nurse with three years' experience in another city. According to Ms. Romero, "Last fall, Ms. Altmann lived with a pusher and overdosed. She was very honest about her drug problem, and I wanted her to make it. I knew she needed a lot of support and trust." Impressed by Ms. Altmann's honesty, Ms. Romero thought that Ms. Altmann should have a second chance.

Ms. Romero had to face the questions: "Ought a nursing administrator allow a nurse with a history of drug abuse to continue to work?" and "How ought a nurse resolve a conflict between her professional obligations and her personal desire to befriend a fellow nurse?" As the Associate Director of Nursing, Ms. Romero has as her primary obligation the provision of safe, effective nursing care of all clients served by the hospital. Clients must be guaranteed that nurses will always be clear-headed and not under the influence of alcohol or mind-altering drugs. On the other hand, as a sensitive and compassionate person, Ms. Romero also recognized her desire to help Ms. Altmann overcome her drug problem. Thus, there was a conflict between

Ms. Romero's professional obligation to maintain standards and her desire to be a friend and helper to Ms. Altmann.

Ms. Romero knew that Ms. Altmann would have daily access to drugs and that consequently she would face extraordinary temptations to steal drugs for her own use. Yet, she also recognized that the length of Ms. Altmann's previous nursing experience and the fact that she had not been found stealing drugs decreased the probability that drug-related problems would interfere with her effectiveness as an RN. Given these reasons, Ms. Romero thought it would be wrong simply to refuse to rehire Ms. Altmann. Therefore, Ms. Romero encouraged her to attend weekly counseling sessions and waited until Ms. Altmann's therapist submitted a written statement that she was able to work safely in a clinical setting before employing her again. Rather than sacrificing either her professional obligations or her personal desire, Ms. Romero apparently found a solution that satisfied both. The case developed as follows:

In order to help as much as possible, Ms. Romero assigned Ms. Altmann to work with a competent and supportive head nurse, where she did well for four months. Then, last week, the head nurse learned that 500 milligrams of Demerol had been signed out but not given to a patient. The head nurse talked with the patient, who was coherent enough to verify that he had not received the drug, and with Ms. Altmann, who admitted she had taken it.

When Ms. Romero met with her, Ms. Altmann said that something had happened that she could not handle. Ms. Romero was disappointed, for she had expected Ms. Altmann to overcome her drug problem "not only for herself as a person but because she was a nurse." Ms. Romero has "higher expectations for people in certain roles." She believed that Ms. Altmann was a good RN who was embarrassed by the difficulty she had caused.

Ms. Romero knows she is obliged to report Ms. Altmann to the State Board of Nurses and that they will discipline her by rescinding her license to practice. Ms. Romero does not want Ms. Altmann to go elsewhere to work where she may steal narcotics and falsify records again; but, because of her personal involvement, it is difficult for her to terminate Ms. Altmann and to make the report.

Ms. Romero now faces the question: "Ought a nursing administrator allow a nurse who has stolen drugs to continue to work?" The law says that nurses as well as other people may not steal drugs. Although it is understandable that Ms. Romero feels a personal loss, since she sincerely wished for Ms. Altmann's success and gave her practical support, the law and hospital policy require that Ms. Romero must discharge and report Ms. Altmann because she has not fulfilled her legal obligations as a nurse. If Ms. Romero believes that Ms. Altmann was unable to control her desire for drugs, she must acknowledge that Ms. Altmann cannot fulfill the demanding responsibilities of a registered nurse. Thus, Ms. Romero must let her go and report her in order to protect clients from possible unsafe care. If, on the other hand, Ms. Romero believes that Ms. Altmann was able to control her desire for drugs but nonetheless *chose* to steal the narcotics, Ms. Romero should still take the same action. Not to punish Ms. Altmann would be to fail to respond to her as a person with the ability to make choices and to assume responsibility for the consequences of her own choices.[17] Finally, Ms. Romero could simply ignore the situation or forgive her for stealing the Demerol. But either of these courses would have a number of undesirable effects: (1) Ms. Romero would be violating the law and thus involving herself in possible legal difficulties; (2) she would be disregarding professional nursing standards; (3) she would be ignoring a strong sign that Ms. Altmann's future clients might be deprived of needed pain-relieving drugs; and (4) she would be contributing to Ms. Altmann's continuing dependence on drugs. These possible consequences make it unacceptable for Ms. Romero—even given her desire to be a helpful friend—either to ignore the drug theft or to forgive it. Therefore, as argued previously, Ms. Romero should let Ms. Altmann go and report her to the State Board of Nursing.

This case suggests two quite different approaches to the basic question of how a nurse ought to resolve a conflict between professional obligations and personal desire to befriend a fellow nurse. When Ms. Altmann's situation appeared merely to be that of a person with a history of drug abuse and no clear threat to provision of safe, effective care, Ms. Romero was able to identify a course of action that appeared to satisfy conflicting claims. At this point the case underscored a suggestion made earlier in this chapter—that it is sometimes possible to select a course of action that allows one to reconcile what may appear to be competing alternatives. At the point in the situation, however, when the case shifted from an episode of drug abuse to a matter of drug theft, professional obligations and legal demands clearly overrode personal desires.

Does the fact that this case turned out badly imply that Ms. Romero's initial response was wrong? No, we think it does not. Sometimes it happens that the right decision in a particular case turns out badly. For example, a few decades ago doctors and nurses appeared to have good grounds for believing that premature infants in respiratory distress needed oxygen-enriched air in order to thrive. What no one knew until later, however, was that excessive amounts of oxygen caused the tiny babies to be permanently blinded. Although given the limits of medical knowledge at the time, the doctors and nurses had conscientiously made the right decision, the results were unfortunate. Presently, with new knowledge and more refined methods of monitoring oxygen levels, this is no longer a problem.

4. Administrative response to conscientious refusal

Nursing administrators—whether directors, supervisors, or head nurses— must decide how best to deal with nurses who disobey orders or rules because of conscience. The following presents such a situation.

5.5 Working in a bureaucracy: special favors

The only hospital in town, small Fairview Memorial, has a pediatric unit of eight beds, which is an extension of the general medical-surgical floor. Jason Campbell, eleven-year-old son of Eric Campbell, a member of the hospital's Board of Directors, was admitted in the morning after a bicycle accident. He had minor surgery, was doing well, and was due to be released the next day. When Hilary Jones, evening charge nurse, learned that someone had ordered a special steak dinner for Jason, she protested. "Everyone should have the same care," she told Beth Otterson, the nursing supervisor. Making sure that a certain child has everything—ordering a special meal, or giving special care, or providing the best nurse—goes against my grain. I think, being the nurse in charge, I should have control over what goes on on the floor." The nursing supervisor told her the decision that Jason was to have a steak dinner had come from the "higher-ups" and so would not be changed. Anyway, she added, the cost of the dinner was small, no one else had to know, and Mr. Campbell would appreciate the nurses' special concern for Jason.

Hilary was not convinced that giving Jason the special dinner was right, and she said that she would lose her self-respect if she gave in and allowed some patients to receive "VIP treatment." Therefore, she explained, she would not serve the meal to the boy even if it were prepared and sent to the unit.

Hilary's position concerning the special steak dinner presents a problem to Beth since she must decide how to respond to Hilary's insubordination. The basic question she faces is: "How should a nursing administrator deal with a nurse's conscientious refusal?"

In order to discuss this case, we must assume that in this hospital the authority to make decisions concerning the many small details involved in nursing care—including meal selection—rests primarily with the unit charge nurse but that ultimately she is under the authority of her supervisor and the nursing administrative hierarchy. Given this assumption, the nurse must follow her supervisor's directives or risk disciplinary action. We must also assume that the unit level nursing staff will support the charge nurse's nursing decision (that is, in this case they will not serve the meal) unless a nursing supervisor intervenes. Beth can choose to respond to the immediate problem of Hilary's refusal by serving the dinner herself, by ordering another person to serve it, or by taking no action to get the meal served. But whether Jason gets the steak or not, Beth has to decide whether to report Hilary for insubordination.

Beth believes that all persons who are insubordinate should be reported and disciplined, so her first impulse is to report Hilary to the Director of Nursing. Beth also believes that she would cease to be a fair administrator if she did not deal with the nursing staff consistently, and she can cite reasons to support her position. If she did not insist that nurses at each level follow through on decisions and commitments made by persons at higher levels in the nursing and administrative hierarchy, discipline would break down. Further, if at a later date she reported another nurse for insubordination, that nurse could charge her with unfair labor practices.

However, a course of action very different from Beth's first impulse results if she recognizes her responsibility to a subordinate who disobeys because of conscience.[18] Therefore, Beth needs first to decide if Hilary's refusal to serve the meal is an act of conscientious refusal. To be recognized as an appeal to conscience (as discussed in Chapter 4, Section 3) the appeal must: (1) be personal or subjective although the moral standards on which it is based may or may not apply to others; (2) follow a judgment of rightness or wrongness; and (3) be motivated by personal sanction rather than external authority. Hilary's refusal passes all these tests; she spoke only for herself; she based her decision not to serve the meal upon her previous judgment that "VIP treatment" was wrong; and she acknowledged her personal sanction—that she would lose self-respect if she served the meal. Once Beth recognizes that Hilary's refusal is based on such an appeal to conscience, she ought to rethink her initial impulse to report her. Having established that Hilary's apparent insubordination is motivated by conscience, Beth must consider a number of additional factors.

Mechanically responding to people who violate certain rules or directives without considering their reasons can lead to injustice, a fact which the legal system recognizes. For example, very often a judge or jury may select from a range of penalties when determining how severely to punish persons who for different motives and under different circumstances have committed similar crimes. In the present case, Hilary's conscientious refusal to serve the special dinner is quite different than if she had refused because she disliked the child. Thus, for a supervisor to be fair in a case of insubordination involving conscientious refusal, the supervisor should take the nurse's reasons into account.

Another important consideration is that a nurse who conscientiously chooses to refuse an order is often representative of the more effective and thoughtful nurses in an institution. A nursing administrator needs to keep these valuable nurses employed in order to provide the best nursing care possible. Further, a hospital nursing organization will not collapse if it allows some room for the exercise of conscience. Hilary's refusal was not intended to undermine the authority of the nursing system. Rather, she was attempting to strengthen nursing service by ensuring that it was fair to all patients. The nursing administration, given this view, has an obligation to support Hilary's independent nursing judgments based on conscientious refusal as long as the resulting actions fall within acceptable, safe practice. Beth should be relieved that Hilary is not going further by publicizing the hospital's preferential treatment.

Most important, since the nursing administration permits and even encourages nurses to make independent nursing decisions in questionable cases, it has the responsibility to try to reduce the risks that nurses must take in making such decisions. In the steak dinner case, a question remains as to what is the right course of action concerning the provision of a special dinner to a child of an influential person. Both Hilary's and Beth's positions have something to recommend them. Hilary's position is that Jason's preferential treatment is unfair to other children on the unit who would enjoy or who might even be helped by a dinner they especially liked instead of having only "regular" hospital food. As the charge nurse, Hilary believes that she is in the best position to assess nursing care needs and that the nursing administration is attempting to override her skills and judgment in such a way that her other patients will not be treated fairly. Hilary's right-based appeal to equality and fairness does not, however, diminish the force of Beth's utilitarian appeal to the possible consequences of preferential treatment in this case. Since Mr. Campbell is in a position to influence the hospital's resources, it is likely that the hospital and especially nursing service will stand to benefit. Thus, there are good reasons on both sides, and the best course in the steak dinner situation is uncertain. Since the nursing administration encourages its nurses to think for themselves, it ought to be reluctant to discipline nurses who make well-grounded conscientious decisions. A possible negative consequence of disciplinary action in this case is that it will have a "chilling effect" on independent thought and judgment among the nursing staff.

In conclusion, if Jason is given the steak, his father will probably learn of the meal. If he is not given the steak, his father will probably not ever know that it was ordered; but some people in the nursing and/or hospital administration will be displeased, including Beth. Since Beth believes that giving Jason the special dinner is in the hospital's best interest, she may decide to serve the steak herself or ask another person to serve it.

Yet, she still must answer the basic question the case raised: "How should a nursing administrator deal with a nurse's conscientious refusal?" As the discussion has shown, the administrator must first recognize whether the nurse's position qualifies as conscientious refusal. Once she has determined that it does qualify, as it does in Hilary's case, she must not decide too hastily for disciplinary action. In determining how she ought to respond, she must consider the reasons in favor of the refusal, the value of thoughtful, conscientious nurses, the capacity of the institution and the profession to allow some latitude for conscience, and the extent to which an indiscriminately harsh response will repress independent judgment. On balance, we believe that the reasons for not reporting Hilary in this case outweigh those in favor of reporting her.

Notes

1. Robert E. Riegel, *American Women: A Story of Social Change* (Rutherford, N.J.: Fairleigh Dickinson University Press, 1970), p. 182; American Nurses' Association, *Facts About Nursing 76–77* (Kansas City, Missouri: American Nurses' Association, 1977), p. 16.

2. Vern L. Bullough and Bonnie Bullough, *The Care of the Sick: The Emergence of Modern Nursing* (New York: Prodist, 1978), p. 192; Joy Curtis, "Final Progress Report: Minority Project in Nursing, 1972–1977, a study related to the admission, counseling, program planning and instruction of minority students who have indicated an interest in nursing," supported by NU 00003-05 ORD 17603 Division of Nursing, United States Public Health Service, Department of Health, Education and Welfare, Michigan State University, 1977.

3. Florence Nightingale, *Notes on Nursing: What It Is and What It Is Not* (J.B. Lippincott: Philadelphia, Facsimile of First Edition, 1859), p. 6; Virginia Henderson and Gladys Nite, *Principles and Practice of Nursing* (New York: Macmillan, 1978), pp. 15–36. Imogene King, *Toward a Theory for Nursing* (New York: John Wiley and sons, 1971), p. 89; Dorothea Orem, *Nursing: Concepts*

of Practice (New York: McGraw-Hill, 1971), p. 41; Martha Rogers, *Introduction to the Theoretical Basis of Nursing* (Philadelphia: F. A. Davis, 1970), p. vii; Joan Riehl and Sister Callista Roy, *Conceptual Models for Nursing Practice* (New York: Appleton-Century-Crofts, 1974), pp. 294–98.

4. Bullough and Bullough, *Care of the Sick,* pp. 231–32.
5. American Nurses' Association, *Facts About Nursing,* p. 5.
6. See Marcella Z. Davis, Marlene Kramer, and Anselm L. Strauss, eds, *Nurses in Practice: A Perspective on Work Environments* (St. Louis: C.V. Mosby, 1975), *passim.*
7. Edythe L. Alexander, *Nursing Administration In the Health Care System,* 2d ed. (St. Louis: C.V. Mosby, 1978), pp. 230–34; See also Thelma M. Dickerson et al., *Primary Nursing: One Nurse-One Client Planning Care Together* (New York: National League for Nursing, 1977), *passim.*
8. Helen H. Burnside, *Perceived Need for Technical Specialists in Nursing Care of Hospitalized Patients* (New York: National League for Nursing, 1974), p. 46.
9. Michael L. Millman and Miriam Ostow, "Summary of Discussion," in Michael L. Millman, ed., *Nursing Personnel and the Changing Health Care System* (Cambridge, Mass.: Ballinger, 1978), pp. 258–59.
10. Myrtle K. Aydelotte, "Trends in Staffing of Hospitals: Implications for Nursing Resources Policy" in Millman, *Nursing Personnel and the Changing Health Care System,* pp. 132–33.
11. Carmen F. Ross, *Personal and Vocational Relationships in Practical Nursing,* 4th ed. (Philadelphia: J.B. Lippincott, 1975), p. 158.
12. Respect for persons can be a principle in each of the four types of ethical theories outlined in Chapter 2, Section 2, goal-based, duty-based, right-based, or intuitionist. The main difference is whether, as a principle within a certain systematic framework, its status is basic, derivative or subordinate.
13. S. I. Benn, "Abortion, Infanticide and Respect for Persons," in Joel Feinberg, ed., *The Problem of Abortion* (Belmont, Calif.: Wadsworth, 1973), p. 99f.
14. R. S. Peters, "Respect for Persons," in James Rachels, ed., *Understanding Moral Philosophy* (Encino, Calif.: Dickenson, 1976), pp. 205–209.
15. Margaret Adams, "The Compassion Trap," in Vivian Gornick and Barbara K. Moran, eds., *Women in Sexist Society: Studies in Power and Powerlessness* (New York: New American Library, 1971), pp. 555–75.
16. Joann Ashley, *Hospitals, Paternalism, and the Role of the Nurse* (New York: Columbia University, Teachers College Press, 1976), pp. 16–18.
17. Herbert Morris, "Persons and Punishment," in James Rachels, ed., *Understanding Moral Philosophy* (Encino, Calif.: Dickenson, 1976), pp. 210–27.
18. See Ronald Dworkin, *Taking Rights Seriously* (Cambridge, Mass.: Harvard University Press, 1977), pp. 206–22.

6

Personal Responsibility for Institutional and Public Policy

1. The scope of individual responsibility

Up to this point we have been discussing ethical issues that involve identifiable individuals; ethical inquiry, however, may lead us beyond specific individuals to social structures. For what reasons, if any, do ethical considerations require us to identify faults in social structures and then attempt to remedy them?

6.1 Short-staffed in ICU

Last weekend, staff nurse Andrea Moore, who works in ICU, felt she was not able to give patients the kind of care, including frequent enough observations, that she should provide because the unit was short-staffed. After she told the charge nurse that she had too much to do, the charge nurse called the supervisor whose answer was to "make do." Andrea knew then that she had to handle the situation as best she could and leave low priority work undone. One of her patients was on a respirator and required numerous treatments, including IVs. Another man had an aortic aneurysm and two women had had major surgery. When the physician ordered a variety of treatments and observations, including some scheduled for every fifteen minutes, the charge nurse again called the supervisor for more help and again was told to make do with the staff on duty. Andrea found herself thinking, "I should be doing this and checking that but I don't have the time." When one of the physicians told Andrea that he needed help with another treatment, she exploded angrily, "We just can't do it! We are really short-staffed today." She was sorry immediately for her outburst, but she remembers thinking, "I don't want to hear him yelling at me because I should be doing something and I am doing the most I can."

At the end of the shift Andrea went home upset, knowing that she should have done more, and could have, if there had been better staffing. The longer she thought about the day, the more she came to believe that no one understood the situation. The physicians wanted done what they judged needed to be done, the nursing supervisor believed the nurses could make do, and Andrea was left to juggle details. Andrea thought that the doctors and the supervisors seemed to be doing their best, but still everything was a mess.

Andrea's exasperation and distress arise not only from the way she is limited by the hospital's allocation of resources to providing substandard nursing care but also probably from an apprehension that the situation may be beyond her—or perhaps anyone's—control. What may underlie her feeling of hopelessness is the sense that her difficulties are the result, not so much of the deliberate intentions and choices of identifiable individuals, but rather of the impersonal and complex interplay of social forces and structures—"the system."

This situation, of course, is not unique to nursing. Yet it does raise the question, to what extent and for what reasons should Andrea try, first, to determine why the ICU is chronically understaffed and, second, to do something about it?

According to the rules and principles defining the institution of nursing, nurses have social as well as individual obligations. The Code of the International Council of Nurses states that "The nurse shares with other citizens the responsibility for initiating and supporting action to meet the health and social needs of the public" (Appendix A); and Point 9 of the Code of the American Nurses' Association maintains that "The Nurse participates in the profession's efforts to establish and maintain conditions of employment conducive to high quality nursing care" (Appendix B). Although the codes do not argue for these claims, we believe that their concern with questions of social as well as individual ethics is well grounded.

Generally, an obligation to provide a certain level of care to individuals entails as a corollary an obligation to take steps to insure that conditions exist for providing that level of care. As John Ladd has pointed out,

A parent's responsibility for the health or welfare of his child implies, for example, that if he does not have the power (e.g., the money) or the competence (e.g., the knowledge) to take care of his child, he should forthwith try to get them. There is no reason to think that the same logic does not apply to participants in a social process: if they do not have the power or competence to fulfill their responsibilities they should take all the necessary steps to obtain them. [1]

In the nursing context, this line of reasoning implies that in Case 6.1 Andrea's obligation to provide standard nursing care to the patients to whom she is assigned entails a further obligation to make an effort to identify the source of the staffing problem and to correct it. Since the grounds of this obligation are not limited to nursing, however, it is important to note that the responsibility in question does not fall solely on Andrea's shoulders. Nursing supervisors, physicians, hospital administrators, and possibly others are also obligated in various, and in some cases greater, degrees to attend to the problem. But if they do not appear to be fulfilling their responsibilities, Andrea's responsibility, though perhaps not increased, is not thereby diminished. She still owes it to her patients to make reasonable efforts to determine why the ICU is chronically understaffed and then to try to do something about it.

If we agree that Andrea has a prima facie obligation to try to remedy the situation and that the situation may involve a complex network of social structures, how does she discharge her obligation? Before addressing this question directly, we must explain what we mean by "social structures."

Social structures include organizations (like hospitals), institutions (like medicine and nursing), and practices (like fee-for-service or third-party-payment modes of financing health care). A particular combination of social structures dealing with a more or less restricted set of goods may be called a "system," as, for example, the health care system.

Following Etzioni, we take *organizations* to be "social units (or human groupings) deliberately constructed and reconstructed to seek specific goals."[2] Standard examples are corporations, armies, schools, churches, prisons, and hospitals. Organizations differ from the other kinds of social structures in having more explicit goal-directedness and greater control over their nature and destiny. The prominent characteristics of organizations are: (a) explicit divisions of labor and power; (b) one or more power centers that control members' efforts and direct them towards the organization's goals; and (c) substitution of personnel.

Institutions, as we understand them, are social structures that differ from organizations principally in having less control over their nature and destiny.

Examples of institutions are property, marriage, the family, nursing, and medicine. Social institutions fulfill certain functions in society and they are characterized by certain rules that fix roles and determine relationships in particular contexts. Nursing and medicine, for example, circumscribe different roles for patients and providers and presume different though complementary roles for nurses and doctors. Finally, although institutions as such do not exert direct control over their own nature and destiny, organizations may be created and maintained that are aimed at shaping and strengthening particular institutions. Thus, the American Nurses' Association and the American Medical Association, both organizations, have as their goal the shaping and strengthening of the institutions of nursing and medicine, respectively.

Practices are made up of rules that coordinate and regulate behavior in determinable ways. Common examples are the "-isms," like racism, sexism, capitalism, and socialism. Controversies over the merits of capitalism and socialism are mirrored in health care controversies over the merits of fee-for-service vs. a nationalized health service. Practices often involve and relate different institutions and can be supported or opposed by various organizations. For our purposes, what is important about practices is that, like organizations and institutions, they explain various patterns of human behavior.

If we are to understand, for example, why the ICU in Case 6.1 was repeatedly short-staffed, we must try to identify, first, the organizational causes of this state of affairs and, if necessary, the extent to which the conduct of the organization in question—the hospital—is itself restricted by social institutions and practices. If it turns out that the actions of the organization are restricted by certain institutions and that the institutions are, in turn, limited by certain practices, then the organization can be fully understood only in terms of its role within the practices. In this event, by placing the action of the organization (e.g., hospital) within the context of a practice (e.g., fee-for-service or third-party payment for health care) we obtain a deeper understanding of its conduct and are, as a result, in a position to intervene more effectively (perhaps by joining or forming an organization to do so.)

Returning to Case 6.1 and Andrea's obligation to make some effort to identify the source of the problem and to correct it, we suggest the following. Since our concern is not simply that nurses be able to explain situations such as Andrea's, but that they be able also to help change them, a helpful rule of thumb is to examine the *most alterable* possibilities first. In Andrea's case this means restricting her initial inquiry to the hospital and to its suborganizations, such as the nursing service. In discussions with the nursing administration, Andrea could explore alternatives based upon nursing management programs as well as methods to increase employee satisfaction in health care.[3] If that fails, she could then enlist the support and expertise of another organization, such as her state nursing association. The next step, if the problem is rooted in the "practices" governing the distribution and financing of health care, might be to become politically active at the local, state, or federal level.[4]

Apart from these schematic rules of thumb, Andrea should also be sensitive to the detailed history of the situation and the personalities of those involved. She should recognize that although her efforts may be necessary for a satisfactory resolution of the problem, they are unlikely to be sufficient. Any change in the situation may require the action and resources of nursing supervisors, physicians, hospital administrators, or patients. Thus Andrea must be careful not to alienate them by being overly self-righteous or condemnatory. Problems attributable to the unintended or unanticipated workings of complex social structures often require social solutions, and individuals who may be credited with initiating changes are unlikely to achieve their ends without the support and cooperation of others.

2. Institutional policies and strikes

Suppose that Andrea is able to identify the source of the staffing problem but that efforts by nurses to persuade those empowered to correct it are unsuccessful. Would they then be justified in shifting from rational persuasion to a more coercive mode of achieving their ends, such as a work stoppage or a strike? Before examining the ethical implications and possible justifications of such measures, we should briefly review the history and legal status of strikes and other forms of work stoppage by nurses.

Collective bargaining by nurses to change organizational policies has a short history, and the use of strikes and other work stoppages an even shorter one. A movement for collective bargaining began in California during World War II, and in 1946 the American Nurses' Association created an economic security program that endorsed state nurses' associations as bargaining agents.[5] But the 1947 Taft-Hartley Labor Management Relations Act, which specifically exempted nonprofit organizations from recognizing bargaining rights of employees, and the no-strike pledge made by the ANA in 1950, made collective bargaining difficult. Basically, nurses had to depend upon public relations campaigns and moral suasion when negotiating with health care organizations.

The 1960s brought changes. When collective bargaining became a right for federal employees in 1962, civilian nurses employed by the government gained the right to choose a bargaining agent. In 1966, when nurses in the San Francisco Bay area threatened to submit mass resignations after long, unproductive negotiations with area hospitals, the California Nurses' Association revoked the ANA no-strike policy and the nurses negotiated successfully. Nurses also struck successfully in Youngstown, Ohio, during that year, and the threat of resignations or strikes led to successes elsewhere. The ANA repealed the no-strike pledge in 1968, as did the National Association of Practical Nurses in 1969.

In 1974 the federal Labor Relations Act was extended to employees of nonprofit health care institutions so that at long last these hospitals were obligated to bargain with nurses. The law specifies dispute-settling and strike procedures by requiring time limits for notification of intent to modify contracts and, if no settlement is reached, notification of the Federal Mediation and Conciliation Service. Further, the law provides time limits for no-strike, no-lockout periods and requires a ten-day strike or picketing notice. Even though legal dispute-settling and strike procedures exist, not all nurses, as the following case illustrates, agree that strikes, mass resignations, or other work stoppages are appropriate.

6.2 Suggestion for a strike

For the past nine months Alice Byrum has worked part time as evening charge nurse on a twenty-bed surgical floor in Batavia Community Hospital. To help with nursing care she occasionally has three, but usually two, aides and on rare occasions only one. She finds two aides an inadequate number and one impossible. A recent State Department of Health inspection team indicates that the hospital is understaffed. Alice believes that the nursing supervisor and hospital administrators should avoid overloading the floor and hallways with patients and systematically *understaffing nursing personnel. Administrators could tell physicians to stop sending patients when there is no more room in the hospital, and they could hire more aides and nurses.*

Alice is frustrated because, as she says, "You are behind before you start. You can't give adequate care and you can't expect your aides to give good care. It's frustrating knowing the patients aren't getting the care they are supposed to get. I must spend so much time giving meds, making time-consuming rounds with one particular surgeon who insists that I accompany him (the other doctors are more flexible), checking IVs and doing the paperwork that I can't do anything else. The aides do almost all the direct patient care."

Most of the aides rarely get two days off each week because the administration routinely calls them to cover a shortage when they are off duty. Needing to keep a steady job, they comply. Alice, too, has been called to work extra days, but she has repeatedly reminded the caller of her problems in making last minute baby-sitting arrangements. She has also reminded the nursing administration that she stated clearly when she was hired that she wanted to work only two days each week, and she has asked administrators not to call her because refusing makes her feel guilty (which she assumes they want her to feel).

When Alice complained to her supervisor about the overworked nursing staff, the supervisor told her days had 51 percent of the work load, evenings 34 percent, and midnights 15 percent; therefore, the supervisor said, staffing was based on the percentages. Alice, knowing how much work she had to do, replied that the statistics meant nothing. She was offended at being told she had an exact percentage of the work load when she knew she was overworked and had only two aides for help. Alice suspects that her supervisor, a sympathetic listener, never reports her complaints to higher authorities.

Monthly "group gripe" sessions with the hospital nursing staff and nursing administration have brought no results—the same complaints have elicited the same answers. Alice has come to believe that the only solution to the problem is for the nurses to organize and, acting together, stage a walkout strike the next time staffing is hopelessly bad. She has suggested a strike to the hospital evening personnel, who all have the same problems, but no one has supported her. Alice believes that the nurses may "not be the type to do anything, but in any other situation you can bet people would not put up with that kind of staffing. So a strike is not going to happen here. But I am hoping that somehow and in some way . . . ."

Alice believes that both nurses and patients would benefit from a strike. Her two main arguments for a nurses' strike appear to be that it would benefit clients by producing changes that would improve the quality of nursing, and benefit nurses by reducing job stress and requests that they work overtime. In an ideal situation, the nursing care that a hospital demands of its staff does not conflict with the nursing care that nurses believe they should provide. But Alice and the other nurses repeatedly find themselves in situations where they can only provide what they regard as substandard care because of the low ratio of nurses to patients. In Alice's view, the hospital's substandard health care is related to its exploitation of the nursing staff. The question now is whether a strike aimed at correcting the situation is ethically justified.

Deciding to initiate or participate in any form of work stoppage—sit downs, mass resignations, strikes, and so on—is difficult for nurses because of their education and experience as women in a service profession and their inexperience in collective bargaining.[6] Strikes are especially problematic because they amount not only to withdrawing services but also to using the resulting distress as a lever to coerce the hospital or agency into meeting the strikers' demands. Even if efforts are made to provide warning and to staff certain units, such as intensive care, emergency rooms, and a minimal number of general nursing units, the strike will still force some people to wait for care, at the very least inconveniencing them and possibly even harming them. Since nursing strikes by their very nature require nurses to threaten patient services, such strikes bear a heavy burden of justification.

The presumption against nursing strikes, like the presumptions against parentalism, deception, and coercion discussed in Chapter 3, is very strong. Not only may strikes inconvenience and possibly harm clients; they are also likely to backfire. As with strikes by other groups providing vital social services, like police and fire departments, the public is likely to respond negatively when striking nurses seem to be using the sick and infirm as hostages to better their position. Such public perceptions may be detrimental not only to the strikers, but also to the entire profession of nursing. Moreover, even if a nursing strike is successful, lingering acrimony between the strikers on the one hand and hospital administrators, physicians, and the public on the other, may seriously compromise whatever gains the strike achieved.

Although the presumption against nursing strikes is very strong, we do not think that it is impossible to justify a nursing strike. Like the presumptions against parentalism and deception, it can, at least in principle, be overridden by appeal to certain ethical considerations. We turn now to a brief survey of arguments that attempt to justify such strikes.

A. Goal-based arguments

A goal-based argument in favor of a strike aimed at improving chronically substandard care is that while the strike will to some extent inconvenience and possibly harm *presently* hospitalized clients, it will in the long run contribute to significant improvement in the care of *future* clients. This assumes that the aggregate needs of future clients significantly outweigh those of presently hospitalized clients. A nurse choosing to honor obligations to presently hospitalized clients in such a situation would be making a decision based on short-term interests rather than on the long-term effects of perpetuating poor nursing care.[7]

To increase the net balance of good over bad consequences of a nursing strike, those making a goal-based argument could suggest that strikers not withdraw all services to presently hospitalized clients. Obligations to those who would be directly and severely harmed by the strike could be met. Advance warning of an impending strike would allow prospective clients to choose between seeking other sources of care or tolerating delay.

A less direct utilitarian defense of a nursing strike might focus on the long-term benefits to clients of a highly qualified nursing staff with a fairly low rate of turnover. Continued employment of a well-trained staff depends largely on the level of its salaries and working conditions. If these fall well below those offered by other health care organizations or even other occupations, the hospital or agency will be unable to attract and retain good nurses. Thus, nurses may argue that collective bargaining, strikes, and the threat of strikes aimed at improving their working conditions will indirectly, but significantly, benefit clients.

Whether such arguments can justify nursing strikes depends on two factors: the extent to which one accepts the conclusions of a goal-based or utilitarian argument as decisive on such matters, and the extent to which the utilitarian calculations of overall benefits and harms favor a strike. The first issue requires a review of the strengths and weaknesses of such arguments and whether one can accept the implications of adopting utilitarianism in contexts other than this one. The second requires taking into account all of the probable consequences of a proposed strike and not simply those that support one's predispositions. Thus, the long-term gains of a strike must be balanced not only against short-term losses but also against possible long-term losses, such as negative public perceptions and lingering acrimony between nurses and other health professionals.

One final utilitarian argument against a strike merits special consideration. It is often maintained that nursing strikes weaken the profession itself when staff nurses become adversaries of nurses in administrative positions. This objection, however, may ignore the possibility of the profession's being equally weakened by the submission of the rank and file to prevailing practices. Further, it assumes that an adversary relationship, with its conflict and stress, results only in harmful consequences. Such a relationship may, however, also offer certain benefits, such as mutual goal setting and the incorporation of diverse ideas and points of view resulting in improved nursing services.

Therefore, we conclude that utilitarian considerations may, in certain circumstances, support a nursing strike. Whether in any given situation a strike is justified must be determined by careful efforts to predict, weigh, and balance all of its likely consequences. In most cases, however, utilitarian calculations alone are unlikely to override the presumption against a nursing strike because the short-term negative consequences will always be more certain than the possible long-term benefits. Moreover, we have some misgivings about relying solely on utilitarian considerations in this as well as in other settings. Some duties or rights whose justification is independent of appeals to the overall social good may also have a bearing on the question of nursing strikes.

B. Duty-based arguments

At first glance it appears that we can construct a clear and unconditional duty-based argument against nursing strikes. A nurse's primary duty is to provide for the care and safety of her clients. Assuming that the clients in question are present rather than future clients, nurses would have to assure all clients of safe and adequate nursing care during a strike. But this, of course, would undermine the very point of a strike, which is to coerce management into altering its policies by withdrawing nursing services. Therefore, if a nurse's primary duty is to provide for the care and safety of her clients, and the clients in question are present clients, participation in a nursing strike will always be wrong because it requires the nurse to violate her fundamental duty.

This argument presents a plausible alternative to goal-based or utilitarian approaches to the question of nursing strikes. Its strength, however, depends in part on two important assumptions, which may not always be true. First, the argument assumes that the nursing care that would be withdrawn during a strike is safe and adequate. There may, however, be situations when nursing care in a particular hospital or nursing home is so substandard that patients would be better off if during a strike aimed at changing these conditions, they returned home or were transferred to another institution. If, for example, a patient in Case 6.2 were hospitalized for *elective* surgery and the understaffing problem significantly compromised the safety and adequacy of his or her nursing care, nurses would not appear to be violating their duties to this patient by withdrawing their services. On the contrary, the patient would probably benefit from either postponing the operation or having it performed at another hospital. Moreover, it could be argued that *under these circumstances* providing seriously substandard nursing services constitutes a greater violation of the duty to provide safe and adequate care than not providing them.

The second assumption underlying the duty-based argument against nursing strikes is that the clients who would presently be harmed by the strike and the clients who would, in the future, benefit from it are entirely different groups of people. In a number of cases, however, especially where the clients in question are suffering from chronic illnesses requiring periodic hospitalization or nursing home care, those harmed or inconvenienced by the strike and those benefited may be one and the same. In such circumstances, when the benefits appear to significantly outweigh the harm or inconvenience, it could be argued that the nurse's duty to adequately serve the future interests of these clients justifies her taking limited risks with their present interests by engaging in some form of withdrawal of services. There would be no group of innocent victims whose interests would be sacrificed for the benefit of others.

Thus, although duty-based considerations provide a strong presumption against nursing strikes and other forms of withdrawal of services, we have tried to show that there are circumstances under which such actions might be justified within a duty-based framework.

C. Right-based arguments

Nurses, it may be argued, have the same rights as other people, and when employers violate these rights, nurses are entitled to defend themselves. When, for example, nurses are continually required to work overtime because of personnel shortages, are paid considerably less than people performing comparable tasks for other hospitals or agencies, or are denied a voice as professionals in determining the conditions under which they work, they have a right to do what is necessary to improve their situation. If less drastic means fail and nothing short of a strike appears likely to induce the organization to acknowledge their rights, then they have a right to strike.

A difficulty with this argument, however, is that the nurse's right to strike appears to conflict with the client's right to nursing care; and the latter, on the face of it, seems more important than the former. Most clients receiving nonelective treatment would be likely to prefer substandard nursing care to no nursing care at all. So it is unlikely that even clients who sympathize with the nurse's concerns would be inclined to waive their rights to care.

In response we must distinguish *special* from *general* rights.[8] Special rights are conditional, limited in scope, and grounded in special relationships. The rights to repayment of a debt or the keeping of a promise are special rights.

Such rights are conditional in two ways. They are held not against everyone but only against the person who borrowed the money or made the promise; and they depend on the nature of the special relationship between lender and debtor, promisee and promiser. General rights, on the other hand, are unconditional, unrestricted in scope, and grounded simply in being a human being or a person. The right to life and the right to liberty are general rights. The sense in which they are unconditional is the obverse of the sense in which special rights are conditional. Thus, they are held against everyone and depend on no special relationship between rightholder and those who have the corresponding obligation to respect the right. Although only people who have borrowed money or made promises are obligated to repay debts or keep promises to an individual, everyone is obligated not to kill others or restrict their liberty.

The question now is whether the "right to health care" is a special right, a general right, or both. To say, for example, that the right to nursing care is a special right is to say that it is grounded in the special relationship between particular nurses and particular clients. Once a nurse assumes care for a client she acquires an obligation to the client and the client acquires a right against her, just as the making of a promise creates special rights and obligations between promisee and promiser. But in both cases, once the respective obligations are fulfilled, the special relationship is ended and further rights and obligations are contingent upon re-entering into the special relationship. If the right to nursing care is of this kind, then a nursing strike that results in abandoning clients who have already come into the health care system is likely to violate their rights to continued care. If, however, the strike is announced well in advance and makes provision for honoring prior commitments to those already in the system and to those requiring emergency care that can be provided by no other hospital or agency, the extent to which it violates the special rights of clients may be considerably reduced.

But if in addition to such special rights there is a general right to health care that has the same status as the rights to life and liberty, health professionals probably could never justify withdrawing their services. Whether there is such a general right, however, is a matter of great controversy. A right to health care, unlike the rights to life and liberty, is a positive rather than a negative right. Whereas the latter requires only that one not be interfered with, the right to health care requires that the rightholder be provided with certain services. And it may be difficult to satisfy this as well as other positive general rights without coercing others to provide their time or money and thus infringe their negative general rights to liberty and property. For this reason, whether there is a general as well as special right to health care is a matter of much debate. Therefore, an appeal to a general right to health care does not provide a strong basis for opposing nursing strikes, especially when the strikers scrupulously honor the terms of existing relationships with clients and continue to staff facilities providing emergency care that cannot be provided elsewhere.

To return to Case 6.2, we believe that Alice's suggestion for a walkout strike is at least premature and perhaps could never be justified on a right-based theory. First, since the monthly meetings between the nursing staff and administrators are unproductive, a reasonable next step would be for the nursing staff to ask for help from a bargaining agent, such as the state nurses' association, and to negotiate a contract that would address the staffing problems. The 1974 Labor Relations Act obligates the nursing and hospital administration to negotiate with such an agent in good faith. If these collective bargaining negotiations failed, the nurses could then decide whether to strike in support of their demands. Until then, however, a strike is untenable. Without further attempts at rational persuasion, a strike cannot be supported by goal-based, duty-based, or right-based ethical considerations.

If further efforts are unsuccessful, it is possible, though not likely, that utilitarian goal-based reasoning could justify a walkout strike. So too might duty-based reasoning if the strikers could show that current conditions require the violation of basic duties to present clients and that the situation can only be remedied by a walkout strike. On a right-based view, however, the special rights of presently hospitalized clients to even inadequate nursing care are stronger than the nurse's rights or the questionable general rights of the population at large to more adequate care. Indeed, insofar as such strikes require nurses to violate the special rights of those for whom they have already assumed care, it may be impossible to justify any *walkout* strike according to a right-based theory.

3. Public policy: the case of hospice care

In addition to a concern for the policies of the particular organizations within which they work, nurses' obligations to their clients may also require them to participate in shaping public policy. When, for example, an analysis of barriers to adequate nursing care reveals a structural limitation in the health care system, nurses, as well as other health professionals, have a responsibility to help alter it.

6.3 A place to die

Lillian Brown, forty-eight years old and divorced, is hospitalized with terminal breast cancer that has metastasized to the bone. Her doctors have told her that the disease has progressed too far to respond to any more treatment by chemotherapy, radiation, or surgery. Lillian understands this and says that she wants to die at home, to be with her children and grandchildren. Although she is alert, she is very weak, and requires help with meals, dressing, bathing—all basic activities. She is also in severe pain almost constantly. The doctors have promised to "make her comfortable," but she is reluctant to take the medicine that they have prescribed because it "knocks her out." Her married daughter, with whom she has lived since her divorce, works full time and is unable to care for her during the day.

The nurses caring for Lillian are concerned because her needs—to be with her family, to be free of pain, to have emotional support—are not being adequately met in their hospital, which is geared to acute care. Chronic understaffing prevents Lillian's nurse, Norma Shaw, from spending much time with her. In addition, the nurses feel frustrated in not being able to control Lillian's pain. They know that some medications, like Brompton's Cocktail, can relieve pain while allowing the patient to remain alert. Adjusting dosages to the individual patient's response, however, is a time-consuming process. Norma, who is with Lillian throughout the day, is perhaps the best person to make these adjustments, but Lillian's doctor is unwilling to give Norma or any nurse that responsibility. A third problem is that since Lillian is no longer being treated aggressively for her cancer, her insurance company is threatening to stop payment for her hospital stay. She is not a candidate for nursing home placement because of her need for pain control and because she is still experiencing some after-effects of previous chemotherapy. She cannot go home for the reasons cited earlier.

Norma can predict, from past experience, what will happen. Lillian will stay in the hospital because her doctors will order periodic laboratory tests or IV therapy in order to fulfill the insurance requirements for her continued hospitalization. Her basic physicial needs will be met, but her doctors and nurses will have to continue to direct their major efforts to the more acutely ill patients for whom the hospital is geared. Lillian will die here, remote from family and friends, without adequate pain control, and without the emotional support that she and her family so desperately need. Norma and the other nurses, too, will need a source of support to deal with their feelings of loss. [9]

Even if she and the other nurses adequately do their jobs as defined by the structure of the hospital, Norma believes that they will not be providing the sort of care that Lillian needs. Hospitals are generally oriented to acute medical and surgical problems. Medical and nursing staffs are authorized to exercise considerable control over the patient's life in the hospital on the ground that this is necessary to achieve the patient's ultimate goal—cure and the quickest possible resumption of a reasonably normal life. Nursing homes, on the other hand, are designed to provide long-term custodial care for people who are no longer able to take care of themselves. Because persons usually remain in extended care facilities for longer periods of time and do not generally require treatment for acute medical or surgical problems, economic considerations require that staffing be kept to a minimum. Therefore, neither hospitals nor nursing homes are, in their present forms, structurally or temperamentally suited to the special needs of dying persons like Lillian Brown. She requires a form of care expressly designed to respond to the special physical, emotional, and spiritual needs of dying persons and their families. In other words, she needs what has come to be labeled as "hospice care."

The contemporary conception of hospice care was developed first in England and has recently attracted a great deal of interest in the United States. Although there are a number of variations on the basic theme, all forms of hospice care include specialized nursing care, skilled palliative medical care (with emphasis on sophisticated forms of pain relief), and various modes of psychological, social, and spiritual support. The following definition provides a good introduction:

HOSPICE: A program which provides palliative and supportive care for terminally ill patients and their families, either directly or on a consulting basis with the patient's physician or another county agency such as visiting nurse association. Originally a medieval name for a way station for pilgrims and travellers where they could be replenished, refreshed, and cared for; used here for an organized program of care for people going through life's last station. The whole family is considered the unit of care and care extends through the mourning process. Emphasis is placed on symptom control and preparation for and support before and after death, full scope health services being provided by an organized interdisciplinary team available on a 24-hour-a-day, 7-days-a-week basis.[10]

Focused on the needs of individuals with unique sets of values, hospice care allows a person whose life is ending to live his or her last months, weeks, or days in a manner that does not betray the projects, commitments, and way of life that combined to constitute his or her identity as a particular person.

Efforts are therefore made to care for the patient at home for as long as possible.

Ida Martinson and William F. Henry have recently investigated the feasibility of home care for dying children, and their observations are in many ways applicable to hospice care. According to them,

The basic philosophy of this model is that the home is the most appropriate place to care for the dying child and that, because the care is oriented toward comfort rather than cure, parents should be the primary caregivers. Each family is assigned a particular nurse who visits the home when she is needed and is available to the family on a twenty-four-hour basis. The nurse acts as the family's advocate and liaison with the community in general and with the health care delivery system in particular, provides expertise in the technical aspects of the care (such as administration of medications and use of equipment), provides emotional support during the home care and during and after the time of death, identifies community resources that the family needs. While practice varies from nurse to nurse, the nurse almost always acts as an advisor or consultant since the family carries the responsibility for the care of the child.[11]

This account indicates the nurse's importance in both home and inpatient forms of hospice care.

Yet before hospice care can become a genuine option for all those who, like Lillian Brown, may need and want it, a number of changes must be made in the network of organizations, institutions, and practices that combine to form the health care system. As Case 6.3 suggests, the goals of the hospital, the training and aims of physicians, and the practice of paying for health care are all geared to curing illness. Structural changes are necessary if the system is to be more responsive to patients with terminal illnesses who need care without further efforts to cure.

As indicated in our discussion of Case 6.1, nurses have an obligation to make reasonable efforts to alter certain conditions under which they work, and this obligation is derived directly from their obligation to meet the nursing needs of their clients. Norma Shaw, whose efforts to care for Lillian Brown are frustrated by the system, seems to have an especially strong reason to be actively involved in helping make hospice care a genuine alternative for dying patients. But what can she do?

As a preliminary step, nurses and others interested in the development of hospice care can attempt to understand current structural barriers to hospice care. To begin with the most obvious one, there are simply not enough organizations providing this type of care. The basic change needed at this level is either modification of the hospital, so that a wing or unit can be devoted to hospice care, or the creation of free-standing organizations that can focus on the needs of inpatients requiring hospice care. Home care, an essential component of hospice care for people like Lillian Brown, who lives with a daughter who works full time and is unable to care for her during the day, will also require the development of adult day care centers that can offer company and care while family members are at work.

Changes must also be made in the institution of medicine. At least some physicians must be trained and rewarded for caring for dying patients. They must be skilled in various forms of pain relief and be prepared to coordinate and participate in home care. House calls and working as part of a team with nurses, social workers, therapists, clergy, and others must become part of the normal routine for hospice physicians.

Finally, payment practices may have to be modified. Public and private health insurance plans, for example, are currently oriented to hospital rather than home care. Third-party payers are concerned that home care is more easily abused than hospital-based care. Martinson and Henry cite the following reply by an insurance agent to a father's suggestion that his group insurance plan be adjusted to allow him to care for his dying child at home:

the majority of cases where a doctor prescribed confinement at home could easily be prolonged by malingering. I make no implication that a doctor would aid his patient by prescribing home care . . . what I am concerned with is that it would greatly increase the possibility of questionable claims for reimbursement in an area over which the employer and insurance company would have virtually no control.[12]

As Martinson and Henry point out, the question of *control* is critical. Whether control over a dying person's care is to be held by his or her family or by certified organizations or agencies will depend largely on whether practices for financing the care of the terminally ill can be accommodated to home care.

A number of the changes suggested above will require new legislation. Certain modes of pain control, for example, may involve drugs that are presently illegal. Carefully drafted legislation defining and regulating hospice care may be indispensable if public and private insurance agencies are to agree to pay not only for inpatient hospice care but for home care as well. Such legislation will also be necessary to protect dying patients from unscrupulous entrepreneurs concerned mainly about profit margins.

With this in mind, it may seem there is nothing an individual nurse can do. Yet others may well share Norma Shaw's views, and modest but sustained efforts by large numbers of people can be effective. Norma could begin by learning all she can about hospice care, participating in public education sponsored by church groups interested in establishing hospices, and then assisting any local groups that are interested. She could also initiate or participate in efforts of her local nurses' organization to foster hospice care. And she could lobby, either as an individual or as a member of an organization, for changes in the health care system. In Michigan, for example, nurses have had a direct role in drafting legislation to define and regulate hospice care as active members of a Legislative Task Force on Death and Dying. These suggestions, we admit, are broad. But they illustrate an important point: nurses have ways to participate in changing the health care system that will permit the complex needs of clients and their families to be met more adequately.[13]

Inquiry into issues like those raised by Case 6.3 shows again that the nurse's ethical obligations are social and even political as well as interpersonal. If, as we assume, hospice care would allow nurses to meet their obligations to dying clients more effectively, and if there are ways in which nurses can contribute to making hospice care part of the health care system, then nurses have a responsibility to make such contributions as a corollary of their ethical obligation to meet the nursing needs of individuals and their families.

Notes

1. John Ladd, "The Ethics of Participation," in J. Roland Pennock and John W. Chapman, eds., *Participation in Politics* (New York: Lieber-Atherton, 1975), p. 121.
2. Amitai, Etzioni, *Modern Organizations* (Englewood Cliffs, N.J.: Prentice-Hall, 1964), p. 3.
3. See Ruth Barney Fine, "New Responsibilities Call for New Relationships," *Nursing Administration Quarterly* 3 (Winter, 1979), pp. 69–75; for ways of changing organizations by modifying the nurse's professional concepts, see Marlene Kramer, *Reality Shock: Why Nurses Leave Nursing* (St. Louis: C.V. Mosby, 1974) and Marlene Kramer and Claudia Schmalenberg, *Path to Biculturalism* (Wakefield, Mass.: Contemporary Publishing, 1977); for a discussion of "change" and "risk-taking" see Marlene Grissum and Carol Spengler, *Womanpower and Health Care* (Boston: Little, Brown, 1976), pp. 217–65.
4. Beatrice J. Kalisch and Philip A. Kalisch, "A Discourse on the Politics of Nursing," *Journal of Nursing Administration* 6 (March-April, 1976), pp. 29–34.
5. The historical summary that follows is drawn from Philip A. Kalisch and Beatrice J. Kalisch, *The Advance of American Nursing* (Boston: Little, Brown, 1978), pp. 671–82; Vern L. Bullough and Bonnie Bullough, *The Care of the Sick: The Emergence of Modern Nursing* (New York: Prodist, 1978), pp. 205–212; and Catherine Ecock Connelly, Lois Kuhn, Roanne Muldoon, and Nancy Adams

Wieker, "To Strike or Not to Strike: A Debate on the Ethics of Strikes by Nurses," *Supervisor Nurse* 10 (January, 1979), pp. 52, 56.

6. See Kalisch and Kalisch, "A Discourse on the Politics of Nursing."

7. Robert M. Veatch, "Interns and Residents on Strike," *Hastings Center Report* 5 (December, 1975), pp. 7–8.

8. William N. Nelson, "Special Rights, General Rights and Social Justice," *Philosophy and Public Affairs* 3 (Summer, 1974), pp. 410–30.

9. This case was prepared by Maureen O'Higgins Chojnacki, RN, B.S.N., Oncology Clinic, Michigan State University.

10. Sandol Stoddard, *The Hospice Movement* (Briarcliff Manor, N.Y.: Stein and Day, 1978), p. 165f. (An introductory definition prepared by the United States government.)

11. Ida M. Martinson and William F. Henry, "Home Care for Dying Children," *Hastings Center Report* 10 (April, 1980), p. 5.

12. *Ibid.*, 6

13. See Grissum and Spengler, pp. 104–108; and Frances Storlie, *Nursing and the Social Conscience* (New York: Appelton-Century-Crofts, 1970), pp. 195–207.

Appendix A

International Council of Nurses
Code for Nurses
ETHICAL CONCEPTS APPLIED TO NURSING
1973

The fundamental responsibility of the nurse is fourfold: to promote health, to prevent illness, to restore health and to alleviate suffering.

The need for nursing is universal. Inherent in nursing is respect for life, dignity and rights of man. It is unrestricted by considerations of nationality, race, creed, colour, age, sex, politics or social status.

Nurses render health services to the individual, the family and the community and coordinate their services with those of related groups.

Nurses and people

The nurse's primary responsibility is to those people who require nursing care.

The nurse, in providing care, promotes an environment in which the values, customs and spiritual beliefs of the individual are respected.

The nurse holds in confidence personal information and uses judgment in sharing this information.

Nurses and practice

The nurse carries personal responsibility for nursing practice and for maintaining competence by continual learning.

Adopted by the ICN Council of National Representatives, Mexico City in May 1973, and reprinted by permission.

153

The nurse maintains the highest standards of nursing care possible within the reality of a specific situation.

The nurse uses judgement in relation to individual competence when accepting and delegating responsibilities.

The nurse when acting in a professional capacity should at all times maintain standards of personal conduct which reflect credit upon the profession.

Nurses and society

The nurse shares with other citizens the responsibility for initiating and supporting action to meet the health and social needs of the public.

Nurses and co-workers

The nurse sustains a cooperative relationship with co-workers in nursing and other fields.

The nurse takes appropriate action to safeguard the individual when his care is endangered by a co-worker or any other person.

Nurses and the profession

The nurse plays the major role in determining and implementing desirable standards of nursing practice and nursing education.

The nurse is active in developing a core of professional knowledge.

The nurse, acting through the professional organization, participates in establishing and maintaining equitable social and economic working conditions in nursing.

Appendix B

American Nurses' Association Code for Nurses

Introduction

The development of a code of ethics is an essential characteristic of a profession and provides one means for the exercise of professional self-regulation. A code indicates a profession's acceptance of the responsibility and trust with which it has been invested by society. Upon entering the profession of nursing, each person inherits a measure of the responsibility and trust that has accrued to nursing over the years and the corresponding obligation to adhere to the profession's code of conduct and relationships for ethical practice.

The *Code for Nurses*, adopted by the American Nurses' Association in 1950 and periodically revised, serves to inform both the nurse and society of the profession's expectations and requirements in ethical matters. The *Code* and the Interpretive Statements together provide a framework for the nurse to make ethical decisions and discharge responsibilities to the public, to other members of the health team, and to the profession. While it is impossible to anticipate in a code every type of situation that may be encountered in professional practice, the direction and suggestions provided here are widely applicable.

The *Code for Nurses* and the Interpretive Statements are both directed toward present-day practice. Previous *Codes* have been more prescriptive, identifying codes of both personal and professional behavior, describing appropriate relationships with physicians and other health professionals, and identifying certain responsibilities of the nurse as a citizen, an employee, and a person. The present *Code*, while remaining prescriptive, depends more on the nurse's accountability to the client, and, in that sense, represents a change to an ethical code.

The requirements of the *Code* may often exceed, but are never less than those of the law. While violations of the law may subject the nurse to civil or criminal liability, the constituent associations may reprimand, censure, suspend, or expel ANA members from the Association for violations of the *Code*. The possible loss of the respect and confidence of society and one's colleagues are serious sanctions which may result from violation of the *Code*. Each nurse has a personal obligation to uphold and adhere to the *Code* and to insure that nursing colleagues do likewise. Guidance and assistance in implementing the *Code* in local situations may be obtained from the American Nurses Association or its state constituents.

Preamble

The *Code for Nurses* is based on belief about the nature of individuals, nursing, health, and society. Recipients and providers of nursing services are viewed as individuals and groups who possess basic rights and responsibilities, and whose values and circumstances command respect at all times. Nursing encompasses the promotion and restoration of health, the prevention of illness, and the alleviation of suffering. The statements of the *Code* and their interpretation provide guidance for conduct and relationships in carrying out nursing responsibilities consistent with the ethical obligations of the profession and quality in nursing care.

Code for nurses

1. The nurse provides services with respect for human dignity and the uniqueness of the client unrestricted by considerations of social or economic status, personal attributes, or the nature of health problems.
2. The nurse safeguards the client's right to privacy by judiciously protecting information of a confidential nature.
3. The nurse acts to safeguard the client and the public when health care and safety are affected by the incompetent, unethical, or illegal practice of any person.

4. The nurse assumes responsibility and accountability for individual nursing judgments and actions.

5. The nurse maintains competence in nursing.

6. The nurse exercises informed judgment and uses individual competence and qualifications as criteria in seeking consultation, accepting responsibilities, and delegating nursing activities to others.

7. The nurse participates in activities that contribute to the ongoing development of the profession's body of knowledge.

8. The nurse participates in the profession's efforts to implement and improve standards of nursing.

9. The nurse participates in the profession's efforts to establish and maintain conditions of employment conducive to high quality nursing care.

10. The nurse participates in the profession's effort to protect the public from misinformation and misrepresentation and to maintain the integrity of nursing.

11. The nurse collaborates with members of the health professions and other citizens in promoting community and national efforts to meet the health needs of the public.

Appendix C

American Hospital Association
A Patient's Bill of Rights

The American Hospital Association presents a Patient's Bill of Rights with the expectation that observance of these rights will contribute to more effective patient care and greater satisfaction for the patient, his physician, and the hospital organization. Further, the Association presents these rights in the expectation that they will be supported by the hospital on behalf of its patients, as an integral part of the healing process. It is recognized that a personal relationship between the physician and the patient is essential for the provision of proper medical care. The traditional physician-patient relationship takes on a new dimension when care is rendered within an organizational structure. Legal precedent has established that the institution itself also has a responsibility to the patient. It is in recognition of these factors that these rights are affirmed.

1. The patient has the right to considerate and respectful care.

2. The patient has the right to obtain from his physician complete current information concerning his diagnosis, treatment, and prognosis in terms the patient can be reasonably expected to understand. When it is not medically advisable to give such information to the patient, the information should be made available to an appropriate person in his behalf. He has the right to know, by name, the physician responsible for coordinating his care.

3. The patient has the right to receive from his physician information necessary to give informed consent prior to the start of any procedure and/or treatment. Except in emergencies, such information for informed consent should include but not necessarily be limited to the specific procedure and/or treatment, the medically significant risks involved, and the probable duration of incapacitation. Where medically significant alternatives for care or treatment exist, or when the patient requests information concerning medical alternatives, the patient has the right to such information. The patient also has the right to know the name of the person responsible for the procedures and/or treatment.

4. The patient has the right to refuse treatment to the extent permitted by law and to be informed of the medical consequences of his action.

5. The patient has the right to every consideration of his privacy concerning his own medical care program. Case discussion, consultation, examination, and treatment are confidential and should be conducted discreetly. Those not directly involved in his care must have the permission of the patient to be present.

6. The patient has the right to expect that all communications and records pertaining to his care should be treated as confidential.

7. The patient has the right to expect that within its capacity a hospital must make reasonable response to the request of a patient for services. The hospital must provide evaluation, service, and/or referral as indicated by the urgency of the case. When medically permissible, a patient may be transferred to another facility only after he has received complete information and explanation concerning the needs for and alternatives to such a transfer. The institution to which the patient is to be transferred must first have accepted the patient for transfer.

8. The patient has the right to obtain information as to any relationship of his hospital to other health care and educational institutions insofar as his care is concerned. The patient has the right to obtain information as to the existence of any professional relationships among individuals, by name, who are treating him.

9. The patient has the right to be advised if the hospital proposes to engage in or perform human experimentation affecting his care or treatment. The patient has the right to refuse to participate in such research projects.

10. The patient has the right to expect reasonable continuity of care. He has the right to know in advance what appointment times and physicians are available and where. The patient has the right to expect that the hospital will provide a mechanism whereby he is informed by his physician or a delegate

of the physician of the patient's continuing health care requirements following discharge.

11. The patient has the right to examine and receive an explanation of his bill regardless of source of payment.

12. The patient has the right to know what hospital rules and regulations apply to his conduct as a patient.

No catalog of rights can guarantee for the patient the kind of treatment he has a right to expect. A hospital has many functions to perform, including the prevention and treatment of disease, the education of both health professionals and patients, and the conduct of clinical research. All these activities must be conducted with an overriding concern for the patient, and, above all, the recognition of his dignity as a human being. Success in achieving this recognition assures success in the defense of the rights of the patient.

Appendix D

Cases for Analysis

A.1 Refusing the researcher

Matt Burns, head nurse at a large university medical center, was not certain that Dr. Hemphill's oncology research was best for the patients involved. Mr. Burns tried to consider the research from Dr. Hemphill's point of view, which, he reasoned, included concern for the overall results, Hemphill's reputation as an oncologist and researcher, and funding. When Mr. Burns examined the research from his own point of view, he focused on the sufferings of individual patients. He questioned whether the patients should have consented to spend their last months undergoing experimental chemotherapy since the treatments did not seem to help and often made patients sicker. He could support the research and the patients' participation only because he knew there was no cure for them and because he believed that oncology research was vital.

According to Mr. Burns, "Dr. Hemphill insisted on having things his way. The staff nurses on the oncology unit were not paid by him and did not work for him, but he asked us to do many things that I could not okay. For instance, he wrote orders for the nurses to give a certain medication straight IV push, an order that overall hospital policy forbids nurses to carry out. I had to consider what would happen to any of the nurses if they went against the policy, which was designed, I think, to protect them. I also had to be supportive of nursing administration policy in order to remain head nurse." Mr. Burns believed, as well, that his staff wanted him to tell them to follow hospital policy rather than Dr. Hemphill's orders.

When he told the doctor that the nurses could not give the medication straight IV, the doctor asked him to deviate from the policy and not to tell anyone he was doing so. Mr. Burns refused. Dr. Hemphill's solution was to hire his own nurse to give the medication, which created problems for the staff nurses. Adding to the general tension was Mr. Burns's belief that Dr. Hemphill was trying to make his life miserable so that he would quit and the doctor might be able to work with someone he could manipulate. Nevertheless, the doctor's efforts to make Mr. Burns uncomfortable by embarrassing him on rounds in front of physicians, nurses, and patients failed to cause him to resign, and both Dr. Hemphill and Mr. Burns worked to the end of the research period.

A.2 The nursing instructor's dilemma

Margaret Scanson, North Lake Community College clinical nursing instructor, is presently supervising students at Portage City Memorial Hospital. Common practice in the hospital is for nurses not to tell patients whether or not they have cancer, because some doctors prefer that their patients not know. Margaret has suggested to her students that if a patient asks such a question, the student should ask the patient what the doctor has said, and if the patient wishes, should offer to speak with the doctor about the matter.

Margaret assigned a student, Marie Blanchard, to care for Mrs. Bullough, a woman in her early thirties who had a brain tumor. Marie, in the course of being with Mrs. Bullough prior to surgery, observing the surgery, and caring for her afterwards, learned that the tumor was malignant. When Marie arrived the following day to care for her, Mrs. Bullough, who knew Marie had been with her in surgery and the recovery room, immediately asked, "Is it cancer?" Marie was at a loss because the stock answer, "What did your doctor say," seemed such a denial of Mrs. Bullough's need for an answer, and since Mrs. Bullough had good reason to believe that Marie knew the answer, she couldn't blandly say she didn't know. Marie excused herself from Mrs. Bullough and sought her instructor.

After learning that the doctor normally shared a diagnosis of malignancy with his patients but that he would not be available until later in the day, Marie questioned the value of ignoring Mrs. Bullough's concerns. She requested that Margaret allow her to tell the patient or, if that was unacceptable due to her inexperience, that the head nurse or Margaret herself tell Mrs. Bullough that the tumor was malignant. Both Margaret and the head nurse knew the diagnosis and the planned treatment. In addition, both nurses had spent time with Mrs. Bullough during the diagnostic period prior to surgery and probably knew her as well or even better than the surgeon. What should Margaret do?

A.3 Too many medicines

Connie Dellinger, community health nurse for six years, knew that Grace Weiss, a seventy-eight-year-old widow who lived alone, preferred to handle her own affairs. On a previous visit, Connie had encouraged Mrs. Weiss to speak to her doctor about the large number of prescription medications she took routinely. Later, Mrs. Weiss told Connie that the doctor had said she was doing the right thing—she was taking her medicine. Connie was not convinced that Mrs. Weiss had told her doctor clearly that she was taking at least ten different medications. Connie could see, as she had seen before, that the numerous drug containers filled a small cake pan. Connie carefully examined each container and immediately recognized "two different heart medications that did essentially the same thing." Connie now realized that Mrs. Weiss was totally confused about the purpose of her various medications. "It was probable," Connie reasoned, "that Mrs. Weiss was being abused by medication and her doctor didn't really know what was happening to her." However, when Connie said that she would like to check the medicines with the pharmacy, Mrs. Weiss balked; the physician had very recently said that she was doing the right thing. Connie thought that Mrs. Weiss probably did not want her to do anything that might call attention to the fact that she needed help. Nevertheless, Connie chose to ignore Mrs. Weiss's protests, called the pharmacist, obtained a review of the medications, and then called Mrs. Weiss's doctor. The office nurse could hardly believe that such an array of medications had been ordered, but at Connie's insistance she arranged for Mrs. Weiss to show the doctor all her medications. Mrs. Weiss was perturbed at Connie for setting up the appointment, but she agreed to go since the doctor was expecting her.

A.4 Birth control pills

Aretha Washington is a public health nurse in an urban county health department. Among her case load of fifteen to twenty families are high-risk infants and children and potential or actual child abuse and neglect families. During a home visit, Aretha learned that Sheila Long was having leg pains and had been getting refills on her birth control prescriptions without seeing her doctor. Given Sheila's medical history and possible side effects from birth control pills, Aretha thought that Sheila should contact her doctor for *evaluation. Aretha also thought that the physician would take Sheila off the pill and substitute a less effective form of birth control. Knowing Sheila, Aretha expected that Sheila would like nothing so well as the pill.*

Aretha thought, "This woman has to take the pill; I really don't want her to have any more kids. I don't think it's right for children to be born when they are not wanted. Also, Sheila has the right not to have to bear children she doesn't want. But what are the consequences of that? Should she stay on the pill and possibly endanger her life? Should she try something that isn't as effective and possibly have an unwanted child?"

Aretha could see advantages and disadvantages both with Sheila's continuing on the pill and changing to another form of contraception which, though possibly safer, would also be likely to be less effective. Aretha had to decide whether to discuss this problem with Sheila and, if so, whether she should encourage her to opt for one alternative rather than another.

A.5 Sit-down strike

Ronna Smith is one of two registered nurse team leaders in the Pinecrest Care Center north wing, which serves one hundred geriatric patients who require skilled nursing care. Adequate staffing requires thirteen aides on the north wing, but on Sunday Ms. Smith arrived at 6:30 to find she was short-staffed again. For the past four months, she had had an adequate staff fewer than ten days. Lights were blinking, breakfast trays were arriving, and the seven aides scheduled to work announced that they were not staying. To prove their point, they sat in the staff lounge.

The aides were at the breaking point; they were infuriated by minimum wages and the task of caring for one hundred people with only seven or even fewer aides. Aware that they could not do an adequate job and tired of everyone's complaints, they had met repeatedly with the administration but had made no progress.

Ms. Smith called her director, who told her to "try to be a motivating leader"; but Ms. Smith thought, "How am I going to motivate anyone when I feel pretty unmotivated myself?" She knew the patients needed help from more aides than the administration had hired, and she felt sorry for the patients, the aides, and herself. Even while on the phone, she could hear the patients calling impatiently for help. She quickly told the director she must come to the center and, with the other team leaders, attempted to answer the blinking lights and calls for help from the patients.

The director came, and, after failing to convince the aides to return to work, she called the departmental administrator, who finally arrived after almost an hour's delay. After three hours the sit-down strike ended with a promise of time-and-a-half for the day and with another meeting between the aides and administration scheduled for Monday. At that meeting all the aides received a ten-cent hourly raise and the promise that when the north wing was short-staffed in the future, each would receive a five-dollar bonus for the day.

Ms. Smith was not satisfied because she believed that paying more for the same inadequate level of service would not help the patients or the nursing staff. After work on Monday, she contemplated resigning. After Ms. Smith married four months ago, she took the job at the nursing home because she could get day work and no shift rotation. However, she was offered $1.50 less per hour than at the hospital and was told that the nursing home did not pay differentials for weekends or shifts because nurses were hired for the shift they selected. On the other hand, she believes that she has developed professionally in this, her first nursing home job: she has learned much about older people, finds her care of geriatric patients rewarding, likes the responsibility, and works well with the doctors, especially the man who cares for most of the patients. She has learned, however, that few nurses stay for more than a year and that many aides stay less than a week. The nursing director repeatedly hires people as aides who have no prior experience or training, so that consequently the team leaders must teach them. Ms. Smith resents the lost time she has spent on those who have quit after the first day or two of orientation and training. She has talked repeatedly to the nursing director and administrator about the low pay scale for aides and nurses, hiring poorly qualified people, consequent high turnover rates, and detrimental effects on the patients' welfare, only to be told that because the center is new and takes a while to grow, they are sorry but, at present, nurses' wages can not be raised.

Ms. Smith seriously doubts that the short-staffing problem will be re-solved merely because the administration made some concessions to the aides. After seeing how drastically the many helpless patients were affected by even a three-hour sit-down strike (no one was fed until after 9:30), she does not believe that she and the other registered nurse should use a strike in trying to change pay scales and hiring policies. Yet talking has been useless, and if she leaves, some other nurse will take the job and the cycle will only continue. Ms. Smith now wonders whether she would be ethically justified if she joined the aides to exert pressure on an administration that has refused to respond to the nurses' suggestions and complaints but has responded promptly to the aides' sit-down strike.

A.6 Failure to comply

Joan Horner, staff nurse on a general medical unit in a large urban private hospital, and Mrs. Barton, a seventy-three-year-old retired school teacher hospitalized with a diagnosis of congestive heart failure, look upon Mrs. Barton's fluid restrictions differently. Joan sees that Mrs. Barton must stay within restricted amounts of fluid intake, and she tries to control the amount of fluid available to her. Mrs. Barton, who is oriented and talkative, agrees with Joan's explanations, but she drinks fluids indiscriminately, especially when her friends visit. In describing Mrs. Barton, Joan says that "The restrictions are just not important to her, or she doesn't see what fluids do to her. Maybe she doesn't care." After attempting to reason with Mrs. Barton and to understand the reasons for her failure to comply with the fluid restrictions, Joan tried teasing and finally scolding her to gain her cooperation, but without success. Finally, Joan explained to Mrs. Barton's friends the reasons for the fluid restrictions and gained their cooperation in keeping the bedside intake record accurate so that Mrs. Barton could be kept within the fluid restrictions. Nonetheless, Joan wondered whether she was morally justified in acting behind Mrs. Barton's back.

A.7 Removal of tracheostomy tubes

At 7:55 A.M. Mary Kowalski was about to give report when she heard patients yelling, "Nurse, Nurse." She and two other nurses rushed to the room and saw Mrs. Audrey Johnson turning blue. Her tracheostomy tubes, in place a few minutes earlier, were on the table, and she had a large new dressing with an ace bandage around her neck. After they quickly cut everything off and reinserted the tubes, the other nurses stayed with Mrs. Johnson, who was extremely upset, while Mary left to get another set of tubes and ties. As she passed the nurses' station and saw the two physicians who, without informing the nurses, had removed Mrs. Johnson's tracheostomy tubes and applied the dressings, she said, "We're putting the tube back in; she can't breathe." Ms. Kowalski remembers that neither moved and one said, "Oh, she obstructed, huh." When she returned to the room, a very frightened Mrs. Johnson would not let the nurses leave her to attend report until someone else could sit with her.

According to Ms. Kowalski, "After the crisis was over, the two physicians proceeded to chew us out because we didn't know where the obturator was for the trach tube. They missed the point of the whole incident. They didn't tell us they were doing it, and they picked a very bad time because there were only three of us working that night. When we went to report, there was nobody left."

Ms. Kowalski does not want to be someone the physicians can "walk right over," keep ignorant of information important for safe nursing care, or blame when things don't go right. To her, the doctors had just "yanked out the tube" and walked out, expecting that the nurses—being women—"would clean up their mess." When the situation developed into a crisis, they found fault with the nurses over the obturator.

The nurses first told the physicians how they felt and discussed the incident with the assistant head nurse, who was coming on duty at the time, and who is also the otology clinician. A few days later, however, the same doctors did essentially the same thing. In that situation, however, a nurse observed them and informed the rest of the nursing staff. Ms. Kowalski thinks that the incident concerning Mrs. Johnson should be prevented from happening repeatedly. She has talked with her co-workers, "trying to figure out what to do, and the answer keeps coming up as zero."

A.8 A nurse's suggestion is rejected

As charge nurse of a thirty-two-bed orthopedic unit, Ms. Connie Bowles is used to working with nurse discretion medical orders, to asking physicians for particular medications, and to questioning treatments. She thinks her interdisciplinary relationships with physicians are generally good, especially with some of the surgeons who, as she describes them, "are very open to hearing your points." But her relationship with Dr. Olsen is different.

Dr. Olsen was treating Mr. Floyd Trapp for an orthopedic problem when Ms. Bowles asked him to arrange a medical consultation. The doctor who came was Mr. Trapp's general practitioner. He had discontinued Mr. Trapp's hypertension medication earlier, and after seeing him in the hospital, had not reordered the medication. Ms. Bowles continued to be concerned, however, because "Mr. Trapp was still running a fairly high blood pressure plus having some other symptoms." She told Dr. Olsen about Mr. Trapp's continuing problems and asked if he would consider another medical consultant who was associated with the hospital. In response, Dr. Olsen asserted that he was the doctor, that he would take care of the consults, and that Ms. Bowles should take care of nursing matters.

After he left, Ms. Bowles wondered, "Was there another way that I could have said it but didn't? Could I have done it differently?" She had tried, as she usually did with all doctors, "to phrase questions so they would be nonthreatening." Should she try to find another way to get a medical consult for Mr. Trapp?

A.9 A request to be excused

Norma Miller, surgical scrub nurse, has told her supervisor, Sue Taylor, that she absolutely cannot participate in sterilization procedures. The previous week she had been caught by surprise when immediately after a cesarean delivery the physician had proceeded to ligate the fallopian tubes of the young mother. Even though the mother had requested the operation, this did not satisfy Norma since she is strongly opposed to sterilization on religious grounds.

Sue Taylor is unsure how to deal with Norma's request to be excused from future participation in such procedures. On the one hand, she would like to respect and accommodate Norma's religious views. On the other hand, she thinks that doing so would involve a number of problems: juggling staff assignments would be time-consuming and take her away from other duties; other nurses would probably resent what they would perceive to be special treatment; and, given the hospital's emphasis on cost containment, accommodating Norma would require some additional costs without appreciably improving services. (This case was prepared especially for this text.)

A.10 Refusal to begin a research procedure

An eighty-two-year-old woman is referred to the hospital research unit for consideration in a therapeutic research protocol that may improve her physical condition. The research physician discusses the study with the woman and her husband and, as she is interested in participating, she reads over the Informed Consent document and questions the patient afterward to assess her comprehension of the material. The physician is satisfied that the patient understands, and she schedules her for the study.

Two days later the patient arrives on the research unit to begin the study but is confused and unable to remember why she is there or any of the information provided in the Informed Consent which she had agreed to and signed previously.

After talking with the patient, the nurse refuses to begin the infusion and contacts the research physician. She arrives and orders that the procedures begin according to the study schedule, stating she will take the responsibility *for the decision. (This case was prepared by Katherine McGrath-Miller, M.A., Research Volunteer Services Coordinator, Bronson Clinical Investigation Unit, Kalamazoo, Michigan).*

A.11 Confidentiality and an attempted suicide

In a particular metropolitan area, public health nurses employed by the county health department are organized in teams of four nurses. In the field the nurses practice independently, but they arrange meetings to collaborate on difficult cases, such as that of the Cass family. LeeAnn Cass, pregnant at age sixteen, planned to keep her baby after delivery. Her father believed that he could not afford a separate apartment for LeeAnn and that she must, therefore, stay with the family. Mrs. Cass, age 38, feared that LeeAnn's presence in the home—and the baby's—would upset the family, especially LeeAnn's three younger sisters. Mrs. Cass had been having anxiety with each of her menstrual periods and recurrent urinary tract infections.

Susan Statler, a public health nurse and one of several professionals involved with the Cass family, learned that Mrs. Cass had attempted suicide by taking an overdose of Valium within the month that the various professionals had been working with the family. During a meeting of the nursing team, one team member strongly questioned Susan's decision not to report to the physician that Mrs. Cass had attempted suicide with the Valium and pointed out that Susan was not legally prohibited from passing such information on to the physician. Susan did not want to risk alienating Mrs. Cass by breaking her confidentiality unless it was absolutely necessary. She knew that Mrs. Cass's psychotherapist, a psychiatric social worker, was aware of her suicide attempt. Susan had not discussed with Mrs. Cass whether all the professionals involved with her, including the physician, knew of her suicide attempt. One of her colleagues argued that if the physician knew about it he would probably then prescribe fewer tranquilizers as a limited form of protection for Mrs. Cass.

Within a few days, Susan discussed with Mrs. Cass the question of informing the physician about Mrs. Cass's attempted suicide, but Mrs. Cass rejected the suggestion that she herself inform him or that Susan tell him. Mrs. Cass saw no value in doing so and did not want to discuss personal problems with the physician since she was already doing so with her therapist.

Susan and her nursing team never agreed as to the correct course of action and Susan did not tell the physician.

Suggestions for Further Reading

(This list is designed to supplement sources identified in the text. Therefore footnoted works have been omitted.)

1. Philosophical analysis and reasoning

Annis, David B. *Techniques of Critical Reasoning.* Columbus, Ohio: Charles E. Merrill, 1974.

Baum, Robert, ed. *Ethical Arguments for Analysis.* 2d ed. New York: Holt, Rinehart and Winston, 1976.

Beardsley, Elizabeth L., and Beardsley, Monroe C. *Invitation to Philosophical Thinking.* New York: Harcourt Brace Jovanovich, 1972.

Engel, S. Morris. *Analyzing Informal Fallacies.* Englewood Cliffs, N.J.: Prentice-Hall, 1980.

Salmon, Wesley, *Logic.* 2d ed. Englewood Cliffs, N.J.: Prentice-Hall, 1973.

2. Ethical theory

Bayles, Michael D., ed. *Contemporary Utilitarianism.* New York: Doubleday, 1968.

Beauchamp, Tom L., and Childress, James F. *Principles of Biomedical Ethics.* New York: Oxford University Press, 1979.

Brock, Dan. "Recent Work in Utilitarianism." *American Philosophical Quarterly,* 10 (October 1973), 241–76.

Feinberg, Joel. *Social Philosophy.* Englewood Cliffs, N.J.: Prentice-Hall, 1973.

Frankena, William K. *Ethics.* 2d ed. Englewood Cliffs, N.J.: Prentice-Hall, 1973.

Fried, Charles. *Right and Wrong.* Cambridge, Mass.: Harvard University Press, 1978.

Gert, Bernard. *The Moral Rules.* New York: Harper Torchbooks, 1973.

Hare, R. M. *Freedom and Reason.* Oxford: Oxford University Press, 1963.

Kant, Immanuel. *Foundations of the Metaphysics of Morals.* Beck, L. W., trans. New York: The Liberal Arts Press, 1959.

Martin, Rex, and Nickel, James W., "Recent Work on the Concept of Rights." *American Philosophical Quarterly,* 17 (July 1980), 165–80.

Mill, John Stuart. *Utilitarianism.* New York: The Liberal Arts Press, 1957.

Rachels, James. "Can Ethics Provide Answers?" *Hastings Center Report,* 10 (June 1980), 32–40.

Schneewind, Jerome. "Moral Knowledge and Moral Principles." *Knowledge and Necessity.* Royalty Institute of Philosophy Lectures, Vol. 3. London: Macmillan and Company, Ltd., 1979, 255–262.

Smart, J. J. C., and Williams, Bernard. *Utilitarianism: For and Against.* Cambridge: Cambridge University Press, 1973.

Taylor, Paul W. *Principles of Ethics: An Introduction.* Encino, Calif.: Dickenson, 1975.

3. General and reference works

Bandman, Bertram, and Bandman, Elsie L. *Bioethics and Human Rights.* Boston: Little, Brown, 1978.

Beauchamp, Tom L., and Perlin, Seymour. *Ethical Issues in Death and Dying.* Englewood Cliffs, N.J.: Prentice-Hall, 1978.

Beauchamp, Tom L., and Walters, LeRoy. *Contemporary Issues in Bioethics.* Encino, Calif.: Dickenson, 1978.

Behnke, John A. and Bok, Sissela, eds. *The Dilemmas of Euthanasia:* Garden City, New York: Anchor/Doubleday, 1975.

Brody, Howard. *Ethical Decisions in Medicine.* 2d ed. Boston: Little, Brown, 1981.

Clouser, K. Danner. *Teaching Bioethics: Strategies, Problems, and Resources.* Hastings-on-Hudson: The Hastings Center, 1980.

Edwards, Paul, ed. *Encyclopedia of Philosophy.* New York: The Macmillan Company and The Free Press, 1967. See, especially, the following articles:
"Ethics, History of." (Raziel Abelson and Kai Nielsen)
"Ethics, Problems of." (Kai Nielsen)
"Religion and Morality." (P. H. Nowell-Smith)
"Responsibility, Moral and Legal." (Arnold S. Kaufman)
"Ultimate Ethical Principles: Their Justification." (A. Phillips Griffiths)

Gorovitz, Samuel, et. al., eds. *Moral Problems in Medicine.* Englewood Cliffs, N.J.: Prentice-Hall, 1976.

Humber, James M., and Almeder, Robert F., eds. *Biomedical Ethics and the Law.* 2d ed. New York: Plenum Press, 1979.

Hunt, Robert, and Arras, John, eds. *Ethical Issues in Modern Medicine.* Palo Alto, Calif.: Mayfield, 1977.

Ladd, John, ed. *Ethical Issues Relating to Life and Death.* New York: Oxford University Press, 1979.

Mappes, Thomas A., and Zembaty, Jane S. *Biomedical Ethics.* New York: McGraw-Hill, 1981.
Munson, Ronald, ed. *Intervention and Reflection: Basic Issues in Medical Ethics.* Belmont, Calif.: Wadsworth, 1979.
Regan, Tom, ed. *Matters of Life and Death.* New York: Random House, 1980.
Reich, Warren T., ed. *Encyclopedia of Bioethics.* New York: The Macmillan Company and The Free Press, 1978. See, especially, the following articles:
  "Codes of Medical Ethics: History." (Donald Konold)
  "Codes of Medical Ethics: Ethical Analysis." (Robert M. Veatch)
  "Confidentiality." (William J. Winslade)
  "Ethics: The Task of Ethics." (John Ladd)
  "Ethics: Rules and Principles." (William David Solomon)
  "Ethics: Deontological Theories." (Kurt Baier)
  "Ethics: Teleological Theories." (Kurt Baier)
  "Ethics: Situation Ethics." (Joseph Fletcher)
  "Ethics: Utilitarianism." (R. M. Hare)
  "Ethics: Theological Ethics." (Federick S. Carney)
  "Ethics: Objectivism in Ethics." (Bernard Gert)
  "Health Care: Right to Health-Care Services." (Albert R. Jonsen)
  "Law and Morality." (Baruch A. Brody)
  "Nursing." (Teresa Stanley)
  "Paternalism." (Tom L. Beauchamp)
  "Rights: Systematic Analysis." (Joel Feinberg)
  "Rights: Rights in Bioethics." (Ruth Macklin)
  "Truth-Telling: Attitudes." (Robert M. Veatch)
  "Truth-Telling: Ethical Aspects." (Sissela Bok)
Veatch, Robert M. *Case Studies in Medical Ethics.* Cambridge, Mass.: Harvard University Press, 1977.

4. The nursing context

Abrams, Natalie. "A Contrary View of the Nurse as Patient Advocate." *Nursing Forum,* 17 (1978), 258-267.
Advances in Nursing Science, 1 (April, 1979), issue devoted to nursing ethics.
Advances in Nursing Science, 2 (April, 1980), issue devoted to politics of care.
American Journal of Nursing, 77 (May, 1977), Ethical Dilemmas in Nursing—A Special A.J.N. Supplement, pp. 845-876.
American Nurses' Association. *A Case for Baccalaureate Preparation in Nursing.* Kansas City, Mo.: American Nurses' Association, 1979.
American Nurses' Association. *Ethics in Nursing: References and Resources.* Kansas City, Mo.: American Nurses' Association, 1979.
American Nurses' Association. *Human Rights Guidelines for Nurses.* Kansas City, Mo.: American Nurses' Association, 1975.
American Nurses' Association. *Perspectives on the Code for Nurses.* Kansas City, Mo.: American Nurses' Association, 1978.
Armiger, Sister Bernadette. "Ethics of Nursing Research: Profile, Principles, Perspective." *Nursing Research,* 26 (September-October, 1977), 330-336.

Aroskar, Mila A. "Anatomy of an Ethical Dilemma: The Theory and the Practice." *American Journal of Nursing*, 80 (April, 1980), 658-63.

Aroskar, Mila, Flaherty, M. Josephine, and Smith, James M. "The Nurse and Orders not to Resuscitate." *Hastings Center Report,* 7 (August, 1977), 27-28.

Bandman, Elsie L. "The Dilemma of Life and Death: Should We Let Them Die?" *Nursing Forum*, 17 (1978), 118-132.

Barkes, Peter. "Bioethics and Informed Consent in American Health Delivery." *Journal of Advanced Nursing*, 4 (January, 1979), 23-28.

Beebe, Joyce E., and Thompson, Henry O. "A Paradigm of Ethics for the Maternal Child Nurse." *Maternal Child Nursing*, 4 (May-June, 1979), 141-47, 184.

Bergman, Rebecca, "Evolving Ethical Concepts for Nursing." *International Nursing Review,* 23 (July-August, 1976), 116-117.

Besch, Linda Briggs. "Informed Consent: A Patient's Right." *Nursing Outlook,* 27 (January, 1979), 32-35.

Brooten, Dorothy A., Hayman, Laura Lucia, and Naylor, Mary Duffin. *Leadership for Change: A Guide for the Frustrated Nurse.* Philadelphia: J. B. Lippincott Company, 1978.

Bullough, Bonnie, and Bullough, Vern. *Expanding Horizons for Nurses.* New York: Springer Publishing Company, 1977.

Chaney, Patricia S. "Protest." *Nursing,* 77 (February, 1977), 20-33.

Chaska, Norma L., ed. *The Nursing Profession: Views Through the Mist.* New York: McGraw-Hill, 1978. See especially Hoekelman, Robert A. "Nurse-Physician Relationships: Problems and Solutions," pp. 330-35.

Cleland, Virginia. "Shared Governance in a Professional Model of Collective Bargaining." *Journal of Nursing Administration,* 8 (May, 1978), 39-43.

Cleland, Virginia. "Sex Discrimination: Nursing's Most Pervasive Problem." *American Journal of Nursing,* 71 (August, 1971), 1542-47.

Cleland, Virginia. "To End Sex Discrimination." *Nursing Clinics of North America,* 9 (September, 1974), 563-71.

Creighton, Helen. *Law Every Nurse Should Know.* 3d. ed. Philadelphia: W. B. Saunders, 1975.

Curtin, Leah. "Nursing Ethics: Theories and Pragmatics." *Nursing Forum,* 17 (1978), 4-11.

Curtin, Leah. "A Proposed Model for Critical Ethical Analysis." *Nursing Forum,* 17 (1978), 12-17.

Davis, Anne J., and Aroskar, Mila A. *Ethical Dilemmas and Nursing Practice.* New York: Appleton-Century-Crofts, 1978.

Deloughery, Grace L. *History and Trends of Professional Nursing.* St. Louis: C.V. Mosby, 1977.

Donohue, M. Patricia. "The Nurse: A Patient Advocate?" *Nursing Forum,* 17 (1978), 143-151.

Fenner, Kathleen M. *Ethics and Law in Nursing.* New York: Van Nostrand, 1980.

Glass, Laurie K., and Brand, Karen Paulsen. "The Progress of Women and Nursing: Parallel or Divergent?" in Kjervik, Diane K. and Martinson, Ida M., eds. *Women in Stress: A Nursing Perspective.* New York: Appleton-Century-Crofts, 1979, pp. 31-45.

Heide, Wilma Scott. "Nursing and Women's Liberation: A Parallel." *American Journal of Nursing,* 73 (May, 1973), 824-27.

Jameton, Andrew. "The Nurse: When Roles and Rules Conflict." *Hastings Center Report,* 7 (August, 1977), 22–23.

Kalisch, Beatrice J. "The Promise of Power." *Nursing Outlook* 26 (January, 1978), 42–46.

Kelly, Lucie Young. *Dimensions of Professional Nursing,* 3d ed. New York: Macmillan, 1975.

Lihach, Nadine. "San Francisco: Winners and Losers." *Modern Health Care,* (October, 1974), 32–34.

McClure, Margaret L. "The Long Road to Accountability," *Nursing Outlook,* 26 (January, 1978), 47–50.

Mooney, Mary. "The Ethical Component of Nursing Theory: An Analysis of Ethical Components in Four Nursing Theories." *Images,* 12 (February, 1980), 7–9.

National League for Nursing. *The Emergence of Nursing as a Political Force.* New York: National League for Nursing, 1979.

National League for Nursing. *Ethical Issues in Nursing and Nursing Education.* New York: National League for Nursing, 1980.

Nursing Clinics of North America, 14 (June, 1979), 305–82 devoted to the nurse as an agent of change.

Nursing Clinics of North America, 14 (March, 1979), 1–91 devoted to a symposium of bioethical issues in nursing.

"Royal College of Nursing Code of Professional Conduct: A Discussion Document." *Journal of Medical Ethics,* 3 (September, 1977), 115–123.

Silva, Mary Cipriano. "Science, Ethics, and Nursing" *American Journal of Nursing,* 74 (November, 1974), 2004–2007.

Spicker, Stuart F., and Gadow, Sally, eds. *Nursing: Images and Ideals.* New York: Springer Publishing Co., 1980.

Tate, Barbara L., ed. *The Nurse's Dilemma: Ethical Considerations in Nursing Practice.* New York: American Journal of Nursing Co., 1977.

Werther, William B., Jr. and Lockhart, Ann. "Collective Action and Cooperation in the Health Professions." *Journal of Nursing Administration,* 7 (July-August, 1977), 13–19.

Williams, Frank C., and Williams, Carolyn A. "Ethical Issues in Health Care Policy," in Miller, Michael and Flynn, Beverly C., *Current Perspectives in Nursing: Social Issues and Trends.* St. Louis: C. V. Mosby, 1977, pp. 3–13.

Zimmerman, Anne. "Toward a Unified Voice: Individual and Collective Responsibility of Nurses." *Journal of Advanced Nursing,* 3 (September, 1978), 475–83.

Index